Essays in the History of Medicine

Essays in the History of Medicine

Robert I. Levy, MD

Studies in Medicine, History and Culture

Volume 3

Series Editor: David B. Levy, PhD

2018

License Notes

Version 1.0
תשע"ח
2018

ISBN: 978-1720559344

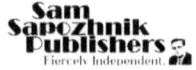

Sam
Sapozhnik
Publishers
Fiercely Independent.

To my parents

Robert I. Levy, MD

and

Ruth S. Levy, ע"ה

Studies in Medicine, History and Culture

Volume One

Music and Medicine

Volume Two

Essays in The History of Nephrology

Volume Three

Essays in History of Medicine

Volume Four

Essays in the History of Allied Sciences

Volume Five

Pierre Rayer's *Treatise sur Les Reins:* A New Translation

Series Editor: David B. Levy, PhD

Preface

Robert I. Levy's first interest in the history of medicine was in high school in 1941 with a paper on the History of Anesthesia. He remembers visiting the Welch Library at the Johns Hopkins Medical School for the first time and entering the stacks in search of some material on this subject. He had the opportunity to visit the Massachusetts General Hospital, and the opportunity of visiting the Ether Dome in the Bullfinch Building where anesthesia was first presented .

In the Johns Hopkins Medical School he had the chance to work part time in the lab of Department of Medicine under Drs. Joseph Lillenthal and Kenneth Zierler This was a wonderful learning experience developing laboratory technique and produced three papers on using Warburg apparatus to study metabolism in rat diaphragm, published in the *Bulletin of the Johns Hopkins Hospital* in 1953 (see bibliography).

While a fellow in the Pharmacology Department of the Johns Hopkins Medical School in 1956-58 with Dr. Gilbert Mudge he worked on the metabolism of diuretics in dogs. This produced two papers published in the *Journal of Clinical Investigation* in 1958 and 1962 (see bibliography).

As a Resident in Medicine at the Sinai Hospital in Baltimore, Dr. Levy dialyzed a patient on a Kolff Twin Coil Kidney with ethylene glycol poisoning in 1958 and wrote up the experience and published in the *Journal of the American Medical Association* in 1960. (see bibliography) This was one of the first patients dialysed in Baltimore before the procedure was performed at Hopkins Hospital, several years later.

Additional review articles were published when Dr. Levy first went into practice of medicine in the Sinai Hospital Journal in 1961 on "Steroid blocking agents as diuretic agents" and in 1962 on "Serum sodium concentration, Facts and Fancy" in *the Indian Medical Journal* in 1962 and "Antibiotics and "Digitalis administration in Uremia" as an editorial in the *Maryland Medical Journal* 13, 35, 1964.

As a result of working in the lab at Sinai Hospital in the Department of Medicine on a NIH grant on Lipids in the Nephrotic syndrome Dr Levy published a paper in the fifteenth *Annual Conference on The Kidney* 1964. (see Bibliography)

In 1964 working with a medical student, Dr. Stewart Fine, who eventually became Head of the Ophthalmology Department at University of Pennsylvania, there was published in the *New England Journal of Medicine* one of the first articles on treatment of pulmonary edema with a then newly released diuretic, Ethacrynic Acid, labeled as a "bloodless phlebotomy."

Early in his practice he published an article in 1966, "Studies in a Patient with Chyluria published in *the Journal of Clinical Nutrition.* Also a study of "Overwhelming Salicylate intoxication in an Adult" published in 1967 in *the Archives of Internal Medicine.* (see bibliography) Both of these papers grew out of clinical presentations, chyluria and salicylate intoxication.

Additional papers were published on the treatment of hypercalcemia with forced saline diuresis and Ethacrynic Acid, a study in dogs and a review of the Clinical Spectrum of Lactic Acidosis, a clinical paper. (see bibliography)

Additional papers on Bromide Detection and Diagnosis of Bromism from the laboratory stand point and a paper on Ectopic ACTH and Hpernatremia were published. (see bibliography)

The presentation of a patient with chyloperitoneum in a patient on peritoneal dialysis presented an opportunity to publish in the *American Journal of Kidney Diseases* in 2001 a paper on studies on this patient and the use of medium chain triglyercide (MCT oil) in this patient. (see bibliography)

Upon retirement from the practice of medicine Dr. Levy began working in the library of the History of Medicine at Hopkins in 2003 and presenting papers on a regular basis to the *American Osler Society* and other venues and forums. With a long history in the practice of nephrology Dr Levy started out on evaluating certain aspects of the History of Nephrology.

The first of these papers on the History of Nephrology was entitled "The Reception in Britain and on the Continent of Richard Bright's *Reports of Medical Cases Linking Dropsy, Coagualable Urine and Small Granular Kidneys as a Clinical Entity- Edinburg, Dublin and Paris*" This paper discusses not only the work of Richard Bright but those who followed, Robert Christian in Scotland, Jonathan Osborn in Dublin, Ireland and Pierre Rayer in Paris.

The next paper *A Garland of Ibids: The use of Footnotes in the Medical Writings of Early Nineteenth Century Authors who Established Bright's Disease as a Clinical Entity"* reviews the use of the extensive footnotes used in the above authors' writings and notes.

Next in the series of papers on the History of Nephrology is a paper entitled, *The Urinalysis as a Factor in the Establishment of the Clinical Entity of Bright's Disease in the Early 19th Century*. This paper discusses the discovery of urea by Von Rouelle and it's further purification and characterization by Fourcroy and Vauquelin who called it *uree*. Berzellus, William Prout, John Bostock, George owen Ress and the Animal Chemists in the Circle of Richard Bright are discussed.

The Animal chemists in the Circle of Richard Bright is a further paper describing the contributions of Berzelius, von Liebig in Germany and Bostock, Prout, Reese, Babington, Barlow and Mr. Tweedies, a medical student and in France, Fourcroy and Dumas on the early study of renal disease.

The Therapeutic Spectrum Available to Those Defining a Newly Recognized Clinical Entity- Bright's Disease discusses the multiple plant sources for medication.

The paper *Pulvis Ipecacunanhae et Opii—The Powder and the Buccaneer—Thomas Dover* further discusses the use of medication available to the early physicians caring for patients with Bright's Disease.

A Conversation Between Two Leeches is a humorous effort to comically discuss leeches in the therapy of renal disease as well as their wide spread use at the time.

A miscellaneous group of four papers followed, the next two having to do with William Osler presented to the Osler society to give a more balanced view of his "therapeutic nihilism."

Sir William Osler's View on Pierre C.A. Louis' Recommendations for Bleeding in Pneumonia.

Sir William Olser —Departure from his Reputation as a Therapeutic Conservative—The Treatment of Bright's Disease.

Sir William Osler's Relationship with William A Marburg and their love of books.

Sir William Osler's Mention of Basham's Mixture.

Colour Indicators in Robert Boyle's Experiments.

Nicholas Monardes Guaicum- Wood from the New World and French Pox.

Dr Levy presented the following paper on *The Doctor and the Newspaper Editor / Correspondence between Logan Clendening, M.D. and H.L. Mencken* at the request of the Medical Department of the University of Kansas Medical School because their founder and benefactor, Logan Clendening, M.D. was known to have been influenced by H. L Mencken in initiating his writing career but little else was known about the relationship. Dr. Levy was a fan of H.L. Mencken, having heard him speak while he was in high school and is a member of the Mencken Society and volunteered to obtain more information on this relationship. The result was this archival search at the Pratt and Goucher College Libraries in Baltimore and the New York City Library and covers not only the occasion of there initial meeting and suggestions of Mencken on writing, but a twenty two year additional follow up relationship that covered a variety of subjects.

"The History of Sinai Hospital" was suggested to by the Chief of Medicine at the Sinai Hospital in Baltimore. While Dr. Levy was born at the Sinai Hospital and was a chief resident in medicine as well as practicing at this hospital for over forty years, the history of the Hospital from its founding in 1863, the third oldest Jewish Hospital in America, was very little appreciated.

"Colour Indicator, Robert Boyle's *Experimental History of Colours and Lignum nephritcum*" was a tale of the Spanish explorer bringing back to the Old World, a wood from a tree that produced a blue color when clear water was placed on it, and was considered by the Mexican Indians and the Old World when it was brought back to Europe in the middle of the 16th Century, as treatment for kidney diseases for over 400 years. Robert Boyle however used it to formulate a definition of acids and bases that was an early advance in modern chemistry. This blue color was also the first known example of fluorescence, a concept not identified until the 19th Century.

Papers in Music and Medicine

Mozart and Medicine at the end of the 18th Century

Johannes Brahms and Dr. Theodor Billroth: A Musical Friendship

Bach and Handel and Cataracts

H.L Mencken and Dr. Logan Clendening: A Friendship

Various Book reviews

The Journal of the History of Medicine and Allied Sciences, History of Nephrology 4: Reports from the Third Congress of the International Association for the History of Nephrology (review), Volume 59, Number 3, July 2004 , pp. 481-483

Introduction

David B Levy

Summers as a child for Dr Levy were often spent in a small coal mining town at the cusp of Western Marlyand and West Virginia, Lonaconing, the birth place of Dr Levy's mother Ruth Bear Levy (zl) daughter of Moses Bear and Linne Eisenberg Bear. Moses was the son of Hartz Bear from Bavaria and Barbeta Jandorf Bear from Wurtenberg,, Germany, while Linnie was the daughter of Gustav and Esther Eisenberg from Hungary. Moses Bear owned a small clothing store in Lonaconing, Maryland.

In Lonaconing Dr Levy as an adolescent worked in the store of his grandfather Moses Bear. After a tiring days of work in his grandfather's local clothing store, at night Dr Levy read by flashlight, classics in the field of the History and philosophy of Science,[1] that sparked interest in this area. In Lonaconing with copies of classics of science purchased with a small allowance, he could not put down such engrossing texts as: Whitehead's *Science in the Modern World*, Tobias Danzig's *Number the*

---

[1] See http://libguides.tourolib.org/philosophyofscience

Language of Science,[2] Newton's *Principia,* Harvey's on the *Circulation of the Blood,* works on Civil War Medicine, Robert Burton's The Anatomy of Melancholy, and Maimonides' *Medical writings*[3] such as those on asthma, poisons,[4] [5]diet, and the commentaries on the aphorisms[6] of Galen and Hippocrates,[7] which have appeared in many translations.[8] If this was not the traditional exposure to Maimonides medical writings by medical students over the centuries,[9] so began a

---

[2] Three more favorite books of Dr. Levy that were recommended to David include Edward Rothstein, *Emblems of the Mind: The Inner Life of Music and Mathematics;* Oswei Temkin, *Ancient Medicine,* David Lindberg, *The Beginnings of Western Science.*

[3] Rosner, Fred , The medical writings of Moses Maimonides, Proceedings (Association of Orthodox Jewish Scientists) 8-9 (1987) 75-91

4 Rosner, Fred, Moses Maimonides' treatise on poisons, Journal of the American Medical Association 205,13 (1968) 914-916

[5] Walker-Meikle, Kathleen, oxicology and treatment : medical authorities and snake-bite in the middle ages, Korot 22 (2013-2014) 85-104

[6] Rosner Fred, The medical aphorisms of Moses Maimonides, Memorial Volume in Honor of Prof. S. Muntner (1983) 6-30

[7] Bos, Gerril, Maimonides' "Medical Aphorisms" : towards a critical edition and revised English translation , Korot 12 [1996-1997] (1998) 35-79. Kottek, Samuel S., Critical remarks on medical authorities: Maimonides' commentary on Hippocrates' aphorisms., Traditions of Maimonideanism (2009) 3-15

[8] Dienstag, Jacob, Translations and editions of Maimonides' medical works : a bio-bibliographical survey, Memorial Volume in Honor of Prof. S. Muntner (1983) 95-135

[9] Ferre, Dolores, Dissemination of Maimonides' medical writings in the Middle Ages., Traditions of Maimonideanism (2009) 17-31.

journey into attempting to better understand the development of the history of science as a process, not a product, not being duped by narrow specialization required today as a result of the technological and bureaucratic revolutions medicine is experiencing. Hopefully the scientists of the future will see the forest for the trees, by the aerial eagle's wings perspective of the long view of the history of science from antiquity to the post-modern condition and become more well rounded, more multi-faceted, and more sensitive to the needs of their patients as human beings. Thus from a young age the thirst for scientific knowledge and a broad perspective animated Dr. Levy' quest for understanding to see the forest for the trees, and apply knowledge gained from historical study to the practice of medicine by expanding consciousness of the place of medicine within a broader historical context.

In courses at Johns Hopkins, Yale, and Harvard Universities, Dr. Levy studied under philosophers and historians of science such as Steven Shapin (*The Scientific Revolution*), Paul Weiss, Arthur Lovejoy (*The Great Chain of Being*), George Boaz (*The History of Ideas*), etc. but mostly Dr. Levy is self motivated as an autodidact to learn on his own. While delving into philosophy and history of science Dr. Levy was also a student of Music Professors Mr. Sklerevsky, Louis Schoub, and Spencer Hoffman.

As Wittgenstein commented, "Thinking and scholarly research does not go on holiday." Ergo upon retirement from medical practice with patients around 2000, Dr. Robert Levy devotes leisure time to not only catching up on playing classical music and learning new pieces, that is a source of love, and visiting museums, with forays into art, literature, history, architecture, and the whole gamut of the Humanities, but also exploring the field of the history of medicine and science that has led to a number of essays in this area. While some may use their leisure in mindless pursuit of cheap thrills, ephemeral pleasures, sporting events, or even fame,[10] Dr. Levy has sought intellectual activity and shared these journeys with fellow historians at various conferences such as *the Osler*

---

[10] In Plato's Lysis and Xenophan's memorabilia we learn from Socrates that the majority of people when given the choice of leisure pursue gashmidik (material) pleasures over intellectual and spiritual virtue. In the *Lysis* Socrates notes that it is common for the many to chase after insubstantial things over friendship. Socrates comments, "All people have their fancies, some desire horses, and others dogs; and some are fond of gold, and others of honour. Now I have no violent desire of any of these things; but I have a passion for friends; and I would rather have a good friend than the best cock or quail in the world: I would even go further, and say the best horse or dog. Yea, by the dog of Egypt, I should greatly prefer a real friend to all the gold of Darius, or even Darius himself: I am such a lover of friends as that." (see Plato, *Lysis, Symposium, Gorgias*, Cambridge, Mass.: Harvard University Press (Loeb classical Library), volume 4, 1925) Here we see Socrates in all the splendor of Socratic irony disparaging those things held by the many to be good in the utilitarian sense. The many have a lack of experience in things beautiful. The Greeks called vulgarity, *apeirokalia*. Socrates' martyrdom in light of a life lived in pursuit of love of wisdom reveals Socrates' beautiful soul. The Lysis goes on to identify the friend with *the Good* and the good with virtue (arete). The above passage cited from Plato's *Lysis* finds correlations with the following from Xenephon's *Memorabilia* where we read, "Just as others are pleased by a good horse or dog or bird, I myself am pleased to an even higher degree by good friends. And if I have anything good I teach it and recommend them to my friends from whom I believe they will be benefited somehow in regard to virtue" (see Xenophon, *Memorabilia and Oeconomicus*, Cambridge, Mass.: Harvard University Press, 1992). It is the excellence of intellectual virtue that is presented in the passage cited from Xenephon's *Memorabilia* where Socrates is said to have shared (literally picked out or selected, from *ek-legein*) enlightening passages from good books. Socrates in the *Memorabilia* continues, "And the treasures of the wise men of old which they left behind by writing them in books, I unfold and go through them together with my friends, and if we see something good, we pick it out and regard it as a great gain if we thus become useful to each other." The man who reports this utterance of Socrates adds the remark, "When I heard this, it seemed to me both that Socrates was blessed and that he was leading those listening to him toward perfect gentlemanship (Kalokagathia)." The greek gentleman posseses the virtues of *megaloprepeia* (magnificence), *megalopsychia* (greatness of soul), and *epiekes* (decent).

Society The *Association for the History of Medicine,* and the American Urological Association (paper on Homer Smith) thus providing a social exchange in intellectual friendship, with other kindred souls who care about such knowledge and its practical applications.[11]

While for Plato and Cicero,[12] intellectual activity is done in community of friendship, for Aristotle

---

[11] See Bos, Gerrit, Maimonides, "Treatise on rules regarding the practical part of the medical art." Ibéria Judaica 4 (2012) 214-248

[12] Unlike Aristotle,intellectual friendship for Cicero is an adequate resting place that need not be surpassed. Cicero finds a *stabilitas* in the friendship of virtue (arete/virtus). When Cicero remarks that *est enim is qui est tamquam alter idem* (for he is, as it were another self) he clearly has Aristotle in mind who refers to the self as the *allos autos*. Laelius asks, "In the first place, how can life be what Ennius calls the life worth living if it does not repose on the mutual goodwill of a friend? What is sweeter than to have someone with whom you may dare discuss anything as if you were communicating with yourself." Cicero makes the analogy that just as good wines improve with age, the oldest friendships ought to be the most delightful. In this matter Rambam follows Aristotle by holding that the highest pleasure is contemplating the attributes of Hashem (in solitude).

intellectual research can be pursued in solitude.[13] Dr. Levy writes the paper in solitude in his small apartment, his goal is to share them with others as John Donne notes, "no man is an island."[14]

Thus Dr. Levy's sharing of his intellectual work at conference is a form of Platonic fellowship, the hard labor of thinking about and writing the papers is Aristotelian. Yet Aristotelian in a Maimonidean key in that Maimonides holds such intellectual activity makes for redemption. Although an

---

[13] Intellectual friendship (a form of Platonic Love) between friends, friendship, in Aristotle is the highest of natural goods. Its being a natural good is apparent in Aristotle's comparison of it to water in the *Politics*. As a good it is said to hold the state together (1155a,1.23). As a good for individuals according to Aristotle "No one would choose to live without friends, even if he possessed all other good things (1155a,5-6). Friendship as a natural good even transcends the good that is justice (*dike*), for "when people are friends they have no need of justice (1155a, 1.26). According to Aristotle the highest kind of friendship is friendship of virtue which is devoted to a good that friends have in common, namely knowledge (episteme). Perfect friendship is the friendship of men who are good and who pursue intellectual virtue (1156b7-8). While utility friends conceive of themselves as profit seekers and pleasure friends conceive of themselves as pleasure seekers, virtue friends conceive of themselves as seekers of virtuous activity. True friendship involves befriending the friend in the name of the good. Friends strive to perfect one another through sharing in discussion and thought (1170b,10-12). When Aristotle notes that "even study is done better with co-workers" he conceives of the *sunergos* who is not a friend in the ideal sense. Aristotle notes that the true friend becomes one's other self united in the quest for truth (*aletheia*) which will ultimately have to be ascended towards alone, even though Aristotle rejects Plato's conception of the forms (*eidos*). Nonetheless the good man is related to his friend as to himself, his friend being a second self or *allos autos* (1166a29-32). Aristotelian friends strengthen one another through mutual care and love in the name of the good which is wisdom, understanding, and knowledge. In that the *eudaemon* life is self-sufficient, the philosopher must leave the magic circle of his truth friends and contemplate the truth in solitude (1177132-4). (see Aristotle, *The Nicomachean Ethics*, Harvard, Mass.: Harvard University Press (Loeb classical Library), 1956). Translations by Martin Ostwald, Richard McKeon, Terence Irwin, and Sir David Ross can also be found.

[14] No man is an Iland, intire of itselfe; every man/is a peece of the Continent, a part of the maine;/if a Clod bee washed away by the Sea, Europe/is the lesse, as well as if a Promontorie were, as/well as if a Manor of thy friends or of thine/ owne were; any mans death diminishes me,/because I am involved in Mankinde; and therefore never send to know for whom/the bell tolls; It tolls for thee.

Aristotelian in many aspects Rambam[15] still would be uncomfortable not only with 1) belief in the heavens as eternal vs. creation *ex nihilo* and 2) not going for the extreme with regards to virtues such as humility and never getting angry as illustrated in Hilchot Deot and the Shemoneh Perakim,[16] and 3) with the Aristotelian appeal to radical solitude that was celebrated much later in history by Emerson and other transcendentalists like Thoreau

---

[15] See http://libguides.tourolib.org/rambam

[16] Rambam's commitment to the traditional Jewish understanding of *creatio ex nihilo* proven by overwhelming textual evidence from Rambam's later writings, that the world was created "after absolute nonexistence," "out of nonexistence," or "not from a thing." That is to say, Maimonides departed from Aristotle in the *Eight Chapters and Hilchot Deot* not only with regard to not adhering to the mean by striving to never get angry and showing that one should be exceedingly humble as Moses was very humble, but also with regard to ultimately rejecting Aristotle's view on creation. One must understand the evolution of Rambam's position on creation in works written besides the *Guide*, including the *Treatise on Resurrection, The Letter on Astrology to the Sages of Montpellier*, The Letter to R. Hisda HaLevy, Medical Aphorisms, and "the revised version" of the fourth of the thirteen formulations of the law in the *Commentary on the Mishnah*. Nothing in the writings of his translator Samuel ibn Tibbon, including the newly edited notes to the *Guide*, suggests that ibn Tibbon considered Rambam's adherence to creationism to be disingenuous. The first denial of this position in the medieval writings of Jewish Averroists, including Joseph ibn Kaspi, Moses of Narbonne, and Isaac Albalag. This denial of creationism ascribed to Maimonides's writings is fallacious, thereby we must be cautious about a Straussian esoteric reading of the *Guide*. While Strauss considers the *Guide* a deeply esoteric work that conceals its religiously complex and problematic Aristotelian ideas from the many, with regard to creationism, Strauss may possibly surround his own position with a body guard of Platonic noble lies.

who retreated outside of community to Walden.[17]
Rambam urges that the life of the mind in pursuit
of wisdom[18]—understanding—and knowledge is a

---

[17] For the Rambam, the Jewish self/ego is only legitimated within a Jewish
community. The Emersonian Romantic notion of individualism and self-making
may be foreign to the medieval halakhic conception of a Jew within community.
While it is true that the Dead Sea Scroll sect retreated into the solitude of the
desert of Qumran; Rabbi bar Yohai and his son lived in solitude in a cave living
on carobs because they were threatened by the Roman government; the Hasdei
Ashkenaz cultivated the virtue of silence in solitude; the Baal Shem Tov lived in
the Carpathian mountains in solitude; and the Kotzker Rebbe retreated into
solitude towards the end of his duration in this world, the Jewish tradition has
always emphasized life in community and association with other Jews. Ten
Jewish men is the minimum halakhic number/quorum required for a minyan.
Life is with people and fellow Jews, making the concept of "self-making" foreign
to mainstream normative Judaism. While it is true certain Tzadikim have
retreated into solitude to work on themselves, and the Musar tradition of Rabbi
Salanter speaks to the need for this kind of self-perfection of Middot, Judaism
has always rejected the solipsistic undertones laden in a modern Romantic
notion of "self-making." For Rambam the prophets sought the solitude of the
desert and wearing rough garments of wool but that was not solipsistic retreat
into solitude as an end for its own sake. Rather prophecy involves annihilation of
the ego what Chasidum call bitul ha-yesh.

[18] Rambam emphasizes the importance of wisdom to guide the messianic age
when he writes, "all the great evils which men cause to each other because of
certain intentions, desires, opinions, or religious principles, are likewise due to
non-existence because they originate in ignorance, which is the absence of
wisdom. If men possessed wisdom, which stands in the same relation to the form
of man as the sight to the eye, they would not cause any injury to themselves or
to others; for the knowledge of truth removes hatred and quarrels, and prevents
mutual injuries." (see Guide 3.2). Rambam's analogy of wisdom to sight is
Aristotelian. In the metaphysics, Aristotle shows that "sight" is the *eidos* of the
material eyeball. Just as the Pythagorean formula shows that the diagonal of an
isosceles triangle is the square root of a2+b2, which has a form, so too do the true,
good, and beautiful have forms. The form of the eyeball is "sight" which has the
form of vision. Emerson, in his essay "The American Scholar," imagines HaShem
Himself to be a "transparent eyeball," a metaphor for an omniscient God.
Aristotle and Rambam prize sight above all the senses. Derrida, in *L'Oreille De
l'Autre*, has seen this emphasis on sight rather than hearing as flawed and
"logocentric." Derrida could point to Rabbi Isaac the Blind (a relation of the
Rabad of Posquires), who was blind but possessed much insight and "vision."
Clearly Rambam, in the wake of Aristotle, would include internal sight as a
reality not to be dismissed, just as Derrida would accredit blind musicians, who
can hear the music they write down in their mind, even though Beethoven was
deaf. In fact many musicians who are composers can hear the music they set
down in notation before it is played in performance.

Introduction 22

noble and redemptive way[19] to devote one's time,[20] and indeed strive for completeness (sheleimuth), and Rambam holds that this activity   in the

---

[19] Rambam views the redemption sub specie *aeternitatis* as the intellectual consummation of the ages, rather than as a redistribution of wealth that the Communists and socialists view reducing everything to class rivalries. Rambam does not view all humans as equal. For example in the *Moreh HaNevukhim*, Rambam dismisses those people who regard anthropomorphisms in the Tanakh literally as inferior to those with a philosophic understanding of such anthropomorphisms. With regards to intellectual virtues, Rambam does not view all as equal and thus with regards to rewards of material benefit these are not to be equal as well. In fact Rambam is with Ralbag that HaShem watches over one with Hashgehah Pratit in proportion to one's intellectual virtues. Rambam rejects the innate equality of people. Einstein is not the equal of most neophytes in physics. Not everyone can achieve the same rank, intellectually. It is not the divisions between rich and poor that will change in the messianic era, but rather a spirit of good will, brotherhood, and peace will come as the result of primitive instincts to fight, envy, and ridicule. While it is true that the hardships of meeting basic needs will be eradicated, for the sages say in Sabb. 30b, "the land of Israel will one day produce cakes ready baked, and garments of fine silk," Rambam sees this as a popular way of expressing the "good times" of the messianic future (Comm. On Mishna, San X).

[20] In the messianic era man will have reached the profoundest knowledge of God, of the exterior world, as well as the complex secrets of his own being. The greatest quest of man will be for God via *Torah Lishmah*'s searching for Hokmah, Binah, VeDaat. Knowledge will be universal. In this sense Paradise is "on this side of the grave," in that intellectual attainment in this life can serve as the foundation for future reward. *Olam Ha-Bah* has already been created although it may be invisible--it is future for those individuals who are destined to enter it (*olam hazeh prozdur li-olam ha-bah*).

messianic era,[21] will be the one preoccupation of the worlds' inhabitants which will be to know-G-d or come closer being with Hashem, via the *sekel hapoel* (active intellect) that once activated, and encouraged by the Philosopher King,[22] allows for

---

[21] Rambam is very sober in regards to his view of the following conditions to be met in the messianic age: no war, no faminine, the lamb (Jews) will not be persecuted by the wolves (other nations), the Temple will be rebuilt with a re-instituted Levitical priesthood, blessings will be abundant, comforts within the reach of all, and the one preoccupation of the whole world will be to know the Lord. Hence Israelites will be very wise, they will know things that are now concealed and will attain an understanding of their Creator to the utmost of the human mind, as it is written, For the earth shall be full of the knowledge of the Lord, as the waters cover the sea (Isa 11:9). With regards to the building of the Beit HaMikdash Rambam writes, "King Messiah will arise and restore the kingdom of David to its former state and original sovereignty. He will rebuild the sanctuary and gather the dispersed of Israel. All the ancient laws will be reinstituted in his days; sacrifices will again be offered" (chapter 11). Rambam legislated that the study of the Korbanot serve as a fitting substitute for the Korbanot until the Beit HaMikdash is rebuilt. Thus one acquires the merit for offering the Korbanot by studying tractates like Birds Nests, Zevahim, Menahot, etc. We must know the details of how to perform the Korbanot when the time is right. Middot, dealing with the dimensions and architecture of the beit HaMikdash, is also essential. Rambam species the following conditions to be met in the messianic era: no war; no famine; the lamb (Jews) will not be persecuted by the wolves (other nations); the Beit HaMikdash will be rebuilt with a re-instituted Levitical priesthood; blessings will be abundant, comforts within the reach of all; and, the one preoccupation of the whole world will be to know the L-rd. Hence Israelites will be very wise, they will know things that are now concealed and will attain an understanding of their Creator to the utmost of the human mind, as it is written, "For the earth shall be full of the knowledge of the L-rd, as the waters cover the sea (Isa.11:9). With regards to the building of the Beit HaMikdash, Rambam writes, "King Messiah will arise and restore the kingdom of David to its former state and original sovereignty. He will rebuild the sanctuary and gather the dispersed of Israel. All the ancient laws will be reinstituted in his days--sacrifices will again be offered. Interestingly the Rambam interprets the verse "the lamb will dwell with the wolf" to mean that Jews (lambs) will not be persecuted by the other nations (wolves), while Abarbanel holds that in the messianic era, wolves will not desire to eat lambs flesh via a change in animal nature. Rambam speculated that the messianic age would dawn in the year 6000 of the Hebrew calendar by interpreting the verse from Tehillim, "a thousand years in your site O L-rd are but a watch in the night" to apply to each of the six creation days in Bereishit." The Rambam warned against such calculation in numerical terms of eschatological fulfillment, and subsequent Hasidic thought such as the Baal Shem Tov asserts that the messiah will come not until the well springs (Torah teachings) are distributed to all four corners of the globe. The messiah, according to one Hasidic parable, is where ever one lets him in.

[22] The messiah or Philosopher King, who will be born in a Davidic family, will trace his lineage back to Ruth. The messiah will not be aware of his royal origin or his priestly mission, and until he has disclosed himself, his family and immediate parentage will not be known (see Zech. 6:12 and Is. 53:2). His destiny will become manifest, however, in due time, and the temporal rulers of the earth will be seized with fear for the security of their thrones and will conspire to overthrow him (*Letter to Yemen*, pp. 6d.). While the mashiah ben Yosef will be assassinated the mashiah ben, David will pass his reign on (Comm. On Mishnah San.). Rambam holds that the messianic state will endure 2000 years and will be an unbroken continuation. The philosopher King will enjoin the world towards intellectual perfection. He will not be an ignoramus, and must excel in learning and wisdom. He will be wiser and mightier than Solomon and well-nigh the equal of Moses in prophetic power. See Hilchot Teshuvah 9.2).

the receipt of knowledge.[23] Rambam's emphasis on the place of intellectual activity as essential for bringing redemption makes Rambam's messianism unique from many forms of messianism described

---

[23] Maimonides, in the Epistle to Yemen (written in 1172), tells the embattled Jews of Yemen, who are faced with forced conversion to Islam, that devoting themselves to rational perfection will prepare the way (or even constitute) the arrival of the messiah--a parallel to the path toward redemption that Maimonides will later lay out in the Guide. Elsewhere in Rambam's commentary to *Perush al ha-mishnah Sanhedrin X*, Rambam notes the various levels of hope beside that of intellectual bliss that many eagerly await: pleasures of Paradise, where all material things of life will be supplied in undreamed of abundance; glories of the messianic state punctuated by remarkable achievements of King Messiah and the independent and opulent position of Israel; joy of resurrection; attainment in this world of physical happiness (*eudemonia*), i.e. bodily health and security, fertility of lands, and abundant wealth; and expect resurrection of dead and eternal bliss in Paradise. Rambam, with regards to resurrection, writes, "[common] people will ask, 'in what condition will the dead rise to life, naked or clothed? Will they stand up in those very garments in which they were buried, in their embroideries and brocades and beautiful needlework, or in a robe that will merely cover the body? And when the Messiah comes, will rich and poor be alike, or will the distinctions between weak and strong still exist?'--and many similar questions from time to time." The sources for an understanding of the redemption, in Rambam, appear in the *Moreh Nevukhim* when he speculates on the theory of the eternity or the destructability of the universe--(II, 29b) *Letter to Yemen*, chapter 10 of the *Perush al-haMishnah Sanhedrin*, and the last two chapters of the *MT Sefer Shoftim*.

in scholarly and popular works on eschatology.[24] The point of note however is that Being in the image of G-d for Rambam means being capable of intellection.[25] If one is blessed with leisure,

---

[24] Joseph Dan's *Ha-Meshihiyut ha-Yehudit ha-Modernit*. Kavka's book is also not a historical treatment that deals with the messiah and messiah movements in their historical context such as Yosef Klausner's *The Messianic Idea in Israel*, Zion Wacholder's *Messianism and Mishnah: Time and Place in the Early Halakhah*, Leo Landman's *Messianism and the Talmudic Era*, Yosef Klozner's *Ha-Rayon ha-meshihi be-Yisrael mi-reshito ve-ad hatimat ha-Mishnah*, Aviezer Ravitzky's *Messianism, Zionism, and Jewish Religious Radicalism*, or Samuel Heilman's *Past, Present, and Future of Jewish Messianism*. It is also not a historical study of false messiah's within the projectory of Jewish mysticism such as Gershom Scholem's *Sabbatai Sevi: The Mystical Messiah*. Neither is it a popular work such as Jerry Rabow's *50 Jewish Messiahs: The Untold Life Stories of 50 Jewish Messiahs since Jesus and How They changed Jewish, Christian, and Muslim Worlds*. Neither is this a book in the biblical teaching of the messiah such as: Joseph Alobaidi's *The Messiah in Isaiah 53: Commentaries of Saadia Gaon, Salmon ben Yeruham, and Yefet ben Eli*, or Robert Wolfe's *The Origins of the Messianic Idea*. Neither does Kavka address the concept of the messiah in sectarian literature of the Dead Sea Scrolls as do treatments of their leader, ha-Moreh HaTzedek, who was a messianic figure as dealt with by John Collins in *The Scepter and the Star: The Messiahs of the Dead Sea Scrolls and Other Ancient Literature* and Craig Evan's *Eschatology, Messianism, and the Dead Sea Scrolls*. collections of primary texts on the messiah, such as Raphael Patai's *Messianic Texts*. Neither is it a scholarly study of the messiah in Aramaic texts such as the Targumim as is Samson Levey's classic. There is much polemic surrounding the controversy surrounding Habad Messianism such as Berger's critical work and more sympathetic "insider" treatments of Chabad messianism in general such as Alter Eliyahu Friedman's *From Exile to Redemption: Chassidic Teachings of the Lubavitcher Rebbe, Rabbi Menachem M. Schneerson and the Preceding Rebbebeim of Chabad on the Future Redemption and Coming of Mashiach* or Jacob Immanuel Schochet's *Living with Moshiach: An Anthology of Brief Homilies and Insights on the Weekly Torah Readings and Festivals*. Berger is an expert in Jewish-Christian debates regarding the messiah such as *Jewish-Christian Debates: God, Kingdom, Messiah* by Jacob Neusner and Bruce Chilton or historical studies of the medieval debates by Haim Maccoby (*The Talmud on Trial*) and Robert Chazon on the medieval debates on the question, "whether the messiah has come," such as that in Paris in 1240 featuring Rabbi Yehiel, Barcelona 1263 featuring Ramban, and Tortosa 1414 featuring R. Yosef Albo. The messiah idea appears from such experts of medieval Latin texts as Berger to Yiddish scholars such as the messiah in Yiddish literature as is Avraham Novershtern's *Kesem ha-dimdumim: apokalipsah u-meshihiyut be-sifrut Yidish*. In the history of ideas Scholem's *The Messianic Idea in Judaism* has enjoyed much popular interest while Sarachek's *The Doctrine of the Messiah in Medieval Jewish Literature*. Sarachek treatment of the understanding of the messiah and messianic age in Saadia Gaon, Rashi, Solomon ibn Gabirol, R. Judah HaLevy, R. Abraham ibn Ezra, Maimonides, Nahmanides, Hasdai Crescas, and Isaac Abrabanel, with an appendix R. Abraham bar Hiyya, has had more of a selective readership.

[25] Rambam understands "glory only in this, in intellectual understanding and knowledge" (*haskel ve-yaddo'a*). For philosophically inclined Jews, this command to know God through studying Torah was expanded to include the requirement to learn the natural sciences and the Greek metaphysical tradition. Maimonides connects this interpretation of the command to study natural science with the command to love-God, when he writes in Guide III:28 that love of God "only becomes valid through the apprehension of the whole of being as it is and through the consideration of His wisdom as it is manifested in it." It is through the *sekel hapoel* that life is redeemed and is the link to God (*hasekel hapoel zeh hakesher bain Adam veHaShem*). In the messianic world this intellectual link or bridge will be made strong and perfect

devoting this leisure to intellectual pursuits is the purpose for which man was created and separated from other creatures. After the Holocaust however, Socrates pronouncement that the "unexamined life is not worth living"[26] needs qualification, for any form of life is worth living and this gave hope to survivors to indeed carry on.

Chalier qualifies being *in the image of G-d* after the Holocaust as a form of affirming one's Judaism, that the Nazis sought to annihilate.[27] Fackenheim's 614th commandment affirms giving the Nazis no posthumous victories, and that can take the form of intellectual pursuits as redemptive, following the guidance of the Rambam on what it means to be *in the image of G-d*, and certainly not politicizing the Holocaust by scapegoating fellow Jews of different sorts, as a theodic reasoning for the leading

---

26 ὁ ... ἀνεξέταστος βίος οὐ βιωτὸς ἀνθρώπῳ *Apology 38a*

27 Catherine Chalier, "Apres La catastrophe: La pensee d'Emil Fackenheim," *Revue de Metaphysique et de Morale* 90:3 (1985), p. 350. Chalier further elaborates, "Ce retour s'inscrit tout d'abord en faux, volontairement et obstinement, contre la certitude impitoyable qu' on peut detruire en l'homme l'image de Dieu, c'est-a-dire l'humanite meme, Puisque c'est sur le people Juif que les nazis voulurent l'effacer a jamais, ce meme people se doit de montrer qu'il n'a pas reussi. En ce sens les Juifs d'apres Auschwitz representent l'humanite quand ils affirment leur judeite et refusent le deni nazi, quand ils respectent, en eux-memes et en leurs freres, ce principe biblique d'un homme cree a la resemblance du divin. Ne faut-il pas meme affirmer que travailler a restaurer cette image- si eprouvee et meurtrie- et temoigner pour elle jusqu'a l'extreme de ses pouvoirs et en refusant le desespoir, se commande de facon encore plus absolue depuis Auschwitz? Et ne doit-on pas garder souvenir du fait que deja, aux heures les plus lugubres, certains trouverent en eux la force de ne pas renier cette image de Dieu?" (p. 351)

Introduction 27

"causes" of the evil of the Holocaust.[28] While the Holocaust may be the break-fissure-caesura-rupture that marks the separation between modernity and post-modernity, it does not change the value of learning lishma (for its own sake[29]) which expresses itself in different forms from

---

[28] Those who regard the Shoah as a consequence of the punishment for anti-Zionism include Rabbi Y.S. Taichtal (see "A Happy Mother of Children," Jerusalem 5743), Rabbi Menachem Emanuel Chartum (see "Reflections on the Shoah", Deot 18, Winter 1961), and Rabbi L. Kaplan (see: Tradition, Fall 1980: 235-48). These three views are the polar opposite of the Satmar Rebbe who saw the Holocaust as resulting from the sin of Zionism itself. See Vayoel Moshe, The Introduction (New York, 1959) and "On Redemption and Ruth", 4:7 (New York, 1967). In Yeshivah circles, the more widespread opinion was that the sin for which the Holocaust was punishment was the Haskalah in general and the way the intellectuals transformed Berlin into their Jerusalem. They cite what was written by the Baal Meschech Chochmath. R. Meir Simcha Cohen in his commentary on Parashat Bechukotai (Lev.26:44), "Yet even then; and before him by the Netsiv in his commentary, The Gate of Israel (Sha'ar Yisrael). There are also some who link the Shoah to "the footsteps of the messiah" (ikavta d'meshicha). Anti-Theodicy rejects these explanations of the Holocaust in God's plan.

[29] See http://libguides.tourolib.org/philosophyeducation

Confucius[30] to Kant,[31] to the Malbim.[32] However in

---

[30] The Confucian *Analects* opens with the statement: "Is that person not a person of complete virtue who pursues wisdom, understanding, and knowledge although others take no note of them?" The word tao in Mandarin Chinese not only means "the way" but "the great learning." The Confucian gentleman who is trained in pursuit of this learning is always graceful and always proportioned in measuring what is truly eternal and of "value", but this value is not of this world, although the Chinese gentleman may live in this world he is not of this world.

[31] The classic formulation of what in Hebrew is called "Torah lishmah", or learning for its own sake, suggests that ultimate learning need not have a material reward in this world and that real learning is motivated by love for truth as a good for its own sake. Thus Kant distinguishes between learning that is an intrinsic good versus learning that confers an external good such as a prize, credit, or material benefit. Plato's Socrates is said to have lived with a love of wisdom (the etymology of philosophy) and as a lover of wisdom desired nothing more than inquiring with his interlocutors in pursuit or quest of the true, the good, the beautiful and the just. Socrates, according to Diogenes Laertus in the *Lives of Eminent Philosophers* is said to have only owned one cloak and a pair of sandals before he was forced to drink the hemlock poison mandated by the Athenian state on charges that Plato clearly holds were unfair, without just cause, and false.

[32] The Malbim's commentary on Proverbs 31 concerning the Aishet Chayil does not take the praise of the righteous woman in strictly material terms. It is according to the Malbim a mushal (allegory) for the life of continuous learning. The Malbim's analysis is preceded by a number of Talmudic passages where the Rabbis praise the life of learning and pursuit of wisdom as the life in pursuit of study of Torah. In baraita de Qinyan Torah appearing in the 6ᵗʰ chapter of Pirke Avot, we find the following praise of the life of learning: Malbim cites, R. Eleazar said: What is signified in the verse, "She openeth her mouth with wisdom, and the Torah of loving kindness is on her tongue." (Prov. 31:26)? Is there a Torah of loving kindness and a Torah that is not of loving kindness? What the verse means is that Torah that is studied for its own sake is a Torah of loving kindness, while Torah studied not for its own sake, but for an ulterior motive, is a Torah not of loving kindness (BT. Suk 49b). In Ned. 62a we learn: "We have been taught: The verse "that thou mayest love the L-rd thy G-d to hearken to His voice to cleave unto Him" (Deut. 30:20) means that one should not say "I will read scripture so that I may be called "sage", "I will recite mishnah so that I may be called "master", I will study so that I may be designated an elder and have a seat in the Academy."" Rather study out of love, and honor will come in the end. R. Eleazar ben R. Zadok said "Do good deeds for doing's sake, and speak of words of Torah for their own sake. Do not use them as a crown to magnify yourself with, or as a spade to hoe with. The foregoing may be confirmed by inference: If Belshazzar who made use of the sacred vessels only after they had been profaned, was rooted out of the world, how much more so by far he who turns to his own use of the crown of Torah, the crown whose holiness abides and endures forever." (Ned. 62a). R. Zadok said, "make them not a crown to magnify yourself with, nor a spade to dig with. Even so Hillel was wont to say, "He who makes unworthy use of the crown of torah shall perish." Hence you are to conclude, "anyone who derives benefit from words of Torah removes his life from the world" (Avot 4:5).

Introduction 29

Rambam,[33] learning lishma, even scientific knowledge, is clearly a form of devotion that makes for redemption[34] and Rambam's harmonization of science and torah was one such redemptive act. For Rambam scientific knowledge is a part of this intellectual activity and the *sekel hapoel* (active intellect) is the link between human beings and G-d.[35] This intellectualism of the Rambam of course is based on the tannaim and

---

[33] Rambam, in the *Shomoneh Perakhim*, writes regarding how to instill in a young child a love of learning. Rambam concedes that most children may be benefited by habituation. For example if a child learns to put a coin in a Tzedakah box they will cultivate the trait of generosity although they may not solve the problem of homelessness. Likewise, a child may be given an incentive to learn by being rewarded with sweets, and indeed, a child whose first encounter with learning the Hebrew alphabet would actually be encouraged to eat letters dipped in honey to gain an appreciation that learning is sweet, a practice that was done at a time when honey was not easily had, and most people's staple diet consisted of unsweetened foods. However, Rambam urges that eventually one should learn not out of incentive (the reward of honey) but out of a love for wisdom. This is deontological ethics. That is to say, one learns not because one will win a car, or another reward. Learning is not entertainment, but as Rambam urged, hard work. *Lifum zarah agrah*, according to the effort is the reward, and thus Rambam's interpretation of Iyov is that this not-bad person was serving Hashem only to receive a reward and avoid punishment. That is to say Iyov was serving G-d for material gain out of fear (yirah). At the age of bar mitzvah the child should stop being motivated to learn out of mere desire to please the teacher for reward and fear of not learning their lessons, but start serving Hashem, through Torah learning lishmah, serving G-d independent of any material reward. Thus the Talmudic ethic of learning, "Talmud torah kineged kulam."

[34] Rambam notes in *Hilkhot Teshuvah* that the crown on the heads of the righteous in the world to come is the wisdom, understanding, and knowledge gained in this world, which is remembered for good by the heavenly court, which metes out the ultimate rewards of basking in the ziv shekhinah before the throne of Hashem. The Rambam warns anyone who "uses the Torah as a spade by which to dig" (i.e. uses the Torah as a means for material reward) that they will be buried by the Torah, for Moshe Rabbenu, when he neither slept nor ate for 40 days or nights on Har Sinai in receiving the supernatural Torah, was like an incorporeal angel without a body.

[35] See Maimonides, Guide for the Perplexed, I.I; "It is on account of this intellectual apprehension that it is said of man: וַיִּבְרָא אֱלֹהִים אֶת-הָאָדָם בְּצַלְמוֹ, בְּצֶלֶם אֱלֹהִים בָּרָא אֹתוֹ

amoraim's praise for *torah lishma* as a noble value.[36]
For Rambam however unlike the mystics, (even

---

36 R. Meir says everyone occupied in Torah for its own sake (lishma) merits many
things. Furthermore, the entire world is worthy of him. He is called re'a; he is
beloved, he loves G-d, he loves humanity, He gladdens G-d, he gladdens his
fellow human beings. It (Torah studied lishmah) clothes him in humility and
reverence and it enables him to be righteous, pious, upright, and trustworthy; it
keeps him away from sin and brings him close to virtue. People benefit by his
advice, counsel, insight, and strength, as it says in Proverbs 8:14,.."mine are
counsel and resourcefulness I am understanding, courage is mine... Torah's
secrets are revealed to him and he becomes like a bubling spring, an endless
flowing river; he is modest, long suffering and he forgives insults; it enhances
and elevates him above all works."
In a baraita, R. Menachem, son of Yose, expounded the verse Proverbs 6:23,
Mitzvah is ner, and Torah ohr. Scripture likens a mitzvah to a lamp and the Torah
to the sun; in order to tell you that just as a lamp's light is temporary, so is the
protection afforded by a mitzvah. However, Torah likened to the sun is to tell you
that just as the sun's light is forever, so is protection of the Torah. And it also says
(Proverbs 6:2) wherever you turn, she will guide you when you lie down
(euphemism for waiting for resurrection in afterlife), she will watch over you,
and when you wake she will converse with you. Rabbi Alexandri said: "He who
studies Torah for its own sake makes peace in the houshold above and in the
household below." Rav said: "It is as though he built the Temple above and the
Temple below" (according to Rabbi bar Yochai the Beit Hamikdash is 18 miles
above har-habayit). Rabbi Yochanan said "He shields the whole world all of it
from consequences of sin." Rabbi Levy said: "He also brings redemption nearer."
In the messianic age, the Rambam notes the one preocupation of the virtuous
will be to learn lishma.
In BT Tanit 7a, we have been taught that R. Banaah used to say, "He who
occupies himself with Torah for its own sake--the Torah he masters becomes an
elixir of life for him. But he who occupies himself with Torah not for its own
sake--the Torah becomes for him a poison."
Mishnah Peah 1:1 states "These ar the precepts that have no prescribed measure.
The corner of the field left for the poor, the first-fruit offering, the pilgrimage, acts
of kindness, and Torah study" which is amplified in BT Shabbat 127a, "These are
the precepts whose fruits a person enjoys in this world but whose principal
remains intact for him in the world to come. They are: honor due to father and
mother, acts of kindness, early attendance at the house of study morning and
evening, hospitality to guests, visiting the sick, providing for the bride, escorting
the dead, absorption in prayer, bringing peace between man and his fellow" and
the study of Torah is equivalent to them all.

Christian mystics like Jacques Maritain[37]),
intellectual friendship, is not a form of asceticism.
Strauss's distinction between Athens [or science]

---

[37] For Maritain the mad boundless love, what he describes in French as *amour fou*
involves giving oneself over totally to God rather rather than the friend or
intellectual companion. The wisdom of the love of friendship has passed into the
realm of *amour fou* when the desire for the good of one's friend is so boundlessly
mad as to involve sacrificing oneself totally for her. According to Maritain when
the limits of sexual passion are surpassed and the soul passes under the regime
of mad, boundless love for God, what Jewish philosophers cal ahavat Hashem,
then the soul has passed to the mystical state. Maritain writes, "the perfection of
human life or the perfection of charity considered in the pure and simple sense,
or under all relations, clearly presupposes the passage to the predominant regime
of mad boundless love for God, or the mystical life." (231) *Amour fou* for Maritain
renounces the lusts of the flesh. This formulation may be due to a linguistic
aspect of Attik and Koine Greek. In Greek the words for love are Agape (love of
G-d), eros (love between men and women), and philia (brotherly and sisterly
love). In Hebrew terms such as Ahavas Hashem (love of G-d), Ahavas Olam
(love of the world), Ahavat Torah (love of torah as an intellectual study) are not
mutually exclusive and are interrelated as there are 70 faces of Torah, and more
than one road to Jerusalem. Athens and Jerusalam in Strauss' formulation
however notes a distinction between the Greek scientific tradition (Athens) and
Jerusalem (religious traditions).

and Jerusalem (revealed religions)[38] also may not do justice to this dynamic of the rationalist and mystic, or what Rav Soloveitchik refers to as "the Halakhic man" as opposed to *homo mysticus* or lonely man of faith. Rav Soloveitchik suggests that halakhic man or the man of reason, and the *homo mysticus* or lonely man of faith, are possibly two aspects embedded in each human *neshamah* although they will manifest themselves differently in different proportions whether one is a Litvish Talmud learner (lomdan), or Chasid caught up in the vibrancy of Hasiduth. However clearly Rambam is unique in offering the paradigm of the rationalist who can reconcile Athens (science) with

---

[38] The distinction between Athens and Jerusalem, is also found in Harry Wolfson and Lev Shestov, to use Athens for Jewish ends, justifying Jewish anticipation of a future messianic era. Strauss writes, "Philosophy in its original and full sense is then certainly incompatible with the biblical way of life. Philosophy and Bible are the alternatives or the antagonisms in the drama of the human soul. Each of the two antagonists claims to know or to hold the truth, the decisive truth, the truth regarding the right way of life. But there can only be one truth."[Strauss further comments, "Philosophy demands that revelation should establish its claim before the tribunal of human reason, but revelation as such refuses to acknowledge that tribunal."[2] Within Strauss's the following oppositions reign between Athens/ Jerusalem; philosophy/revealed religions; reason/faith; thinking/action predicated on ethics to change the world; theoria/piety (submission to ancestral good); free quest/obedient love; no sense of having strayed/*teshuvah* and feeling of having strayed from what was first given as a revelation; realism replaces hope but the philosopher gains from living beyond hope because he has no fears/hope predicated on returning to a past Edenic relation with God; God is distant (see Kenneth Siskin's *A Distant God*)/Jewish belief that God acts in Jewish history; philosophy speaks of virtue (*arte*) with knowledge as the greatest virtue/ religions speak of moral action and compassion, mercy, and graciousness as immutable active attributes; good is thinking/good is the messianic age and deeds of righteousness; in philosophy questioning is the piety of thought/in revealed religions questioning is to serve the higher foundation of religious belief; in philosophy the superhuman is internal to the mind after Nietzsche's conception of *the ubermensch*/in revealed religion the supernatural is a function of miracles; after Hume philosophy is skeptical/in revealed religion skepticism is irreverent to faith.

Jerusalem (Torah).[39] However the danger that Rambam understands is that the man of Athens dare not come to see himself as the measure of all things and the pilgrim of knowledge keep in mind that the human intellect is nothing compared to G-d's inifinite wisdom. Thus the reason for Rambam's negative theology.[40] Dr Levy is able to dwell both in Athens (Science) and Jerusalem (revealed religion) and represents a balance of these two aspects of

---

[39] See Herbert Davidson, for whom Maimonides was the supreme representative of a philosopher who sought to bring together in harmony in the Guide, Athens and Jerusalem.["The Study of Philosophy as a Religious Obligation," in *Religion in a Religious Age*, ed., S. D. Goitein, (Cambridges, Mass.: Association for Jewish Studies, 1974), pp. 53-68]

[40] Maimonides' negative theology asserts that predications of affirmative attributes of God are dangerous. It is chutzpadic to suggest that human knowledge can transcend to comprehension of HaShem's knowledge. One comes nearest to the apprehension of G-d only through negation. Thus we posit HaShem is not a body, not ignorant, not finite, not powerless. It is the negation of the privation of the attribute which is best for attempting to comprehend the divine. Socrates anticipated this medieval negative theology when he noted that with regards to God's knowledge he felt like he knew nothing for God's wisdom, understanding, and knowledge is without end. Kabbalists when speaking of HaShem's infinity, employ the term *Ayn Sof*. However the Rambam as a rationalist rejected certain elements of Kabbalah, for instance by forbidding anyone to read Shiur Komah where the measurements of the Deity are given. For the Rambam the proposition, *"Ain lo demut haguf ve-aino guf"* carries with it an Aristotelian subtext where the unmoved mover is also incorporeal. In fact Rambam draws on Aristotle's understanding of the unmoved mover as "first cause" (*tachlit rishonah*) as one of the proofs for the existence of G-d. The logic notes that since the heavenly bodies (moon, stars, planets, etc.) are in motion there must have been a first cause, namely G-d, who set them in motion. This is called the proof from motion, but other proofs such as the proof from design and the ontological proof also exist. Noteworthy however is that while the Rambam draws on Aristotle in certain regards, he rejects Aristotle in significant cases as well such as in the rejection of Aristotle's position that the heavens are eternal, for Jews hold that HaShem created the heavens and earth (see Bereshit). Just as there was a first cause there is a final cause, also God, when the messianic era will be realized on the stage of human history. Negative theology of Maimonides with regards to G-d's negative attributes allow one to posit: His not finite, He is not ignorant, for it would be hutzpah to say we can cognize G-d Himself. The one who created the human eye, can He not hear, the one who created the human ear, can He not hear, and the one who created the human brain, we can never totalize the divine Mind/Nous/Intellectus Illuminatus. The perspective from the wings of eagles, is what post-modern science and medicine needs, not only narrow specialization and expertise that risks becoming myopically technocratic.

inquiry into his soul in a refined and harmonious proportion. Dr. Levy is not just a man of science and medicine but widely versed in the whole gamut of the Humanities.

Anyone who meets Dr. Levy will note immediately Dr. Levy's consciousness of the cyclopic abuse to which science sometimes can fall as viewing its methods as the Protagorian measure of all things. Thus anyone who encounters Dr. Levy will note his complete unpretentiousness and being totally free of politics. His scholarship is aimed to achieve knowledge not agendas. He does not seek power and glory and shuns publicity. Meeting Dr Levy many instantly feel a sense of *bitul ha-yesh* as egocentrism, solipsism, and self referentiality are foreign from Dr Levy's character. Dr. Levy's respect and consideration for the needs of all is a *Kiddush hashem* of *kavod ha-briyut* (respect for God's creations). Qualities of genuineness, wholeness, straight-forwardness, impeccable integrity, commitment to intellectual honesty and truth, makes Dr. Levy an inspiration to all that circulate in his orbit. Also from these essays you will see that Dr. Levy never ventures an opinion without thorough investigation of the subject matter. Yet in Dr. Levy as a quiet and refined self-effacing individual there is a remarkable harmony of intellectual discipline and rigor with a fatherly love for people and community. Dr. Levy's life is free from the dross of two faced political pretention, power, pompous greed, and personal agendas. From Dr Levy's writings you will see an openness with which to entertain and consider multiple perspectives and views. Dr. Levy's character embedded in his life's choice to devote much of the time in his retirement to medical and scientific research in the history of the field is magnanimous while at the same time simple, transcendent yet worldly, old yet- profoundly new, rigorous yet compassionate, multi-faceted yet natural and affirmative, that *in the image of man* is the embodiment of thought, reflection, critical analysis, and breadth of intellectual interests that is exceedingly rare in our day and age of intense over specialization. Thus Dr Levy's character that has managed to bitul ha-yesh (negate egotism) is linked to his sense of the tragedy of bitul-zeman, for time is too preciouis to waste.

With Joseph Pieper, in his book, *Leisure the Basis of Culture*, Dr. Levy has come to see leisure not as a time to be wasted with mindless routine jobs that rob the precious time we hopefully are all lucky to receive from G- d, "to cherish our days," and not waste time (*bitul zeman*[41]), but making leisure into something that must be cultivated as an art form. Transforming leisure into a redemptive mission. To

---

[41] See http://www.h-net.org/reviews/showrev.php?id=10382

make our life as Nietzsche urges,[42] into a work of art, but something natural at the same time. This cultivation of leisure for study of the Humanities works in tandem with the rigorous objective criteria of science, being solidly committed to the scientific honesty that is provided in objective

---

[42] For Nietzsche art is a saving sorceress (heilkundige Zauberin). Nietzsche asserts that art is a metaphysical supplement that makes life bearable. Nietzsche writes, "wenn anders die Kunst nicht nur Nachahmung der Naturwirklichkeit, sondern gerade ein metaphysisches Supplement der Naturwirklichkeit ist, zu deren Uberwindung neben sie gestellt" (Die Geburt der Tragodie, (Stuttgart: Alfred Kroner Verlag,1976), p. 186. Nietzsche recognizes that we need art, the beautiful illusion, the redeeming untruth, the bewitching lie, to endure the false, cruel, contradictory, the meaninglessness of the real. For Nietzsche art is the affirmation that counters Schopenhauerian pessimism. For Nietzsche art has the task to save (erlosen) the eye from gazing into the horrors of the night, and to deliver the subject by the healing balm of shining from the spasms of the agitations of the will. Underlying Nietzsche's thinking that "nur als ein asthetisches Phaenomen das Dasein und die Welt gerechtfertigt erscheint" is the assumption that we have a necessary need for illusion because reality is too terrifying. Nietzsche views the Greek religion as the apex of the power of the artistic impulse when he writes, "Der Grieche kannte und empfand die Schrecken und Entseltzlichkeiten des Daseins: um ueberhaupt leben zu koennen, musste er vor sie hin die glaenzende Traumgeburte der Olympischen stellen" (p. 58). The whole pantheon of of the Greek deities was the Greek's answer to the terror and horror of existence. Nietzsche urges one to make one's life a work of art. Nietzsche is against the degeneration of art whereby the journalist triumphs over the professor in all matters pertaining to culture. Nietzsche writes, "Es gibt keine andere Kunstperiode, in der sich die sogenannte Bildung und die eigentliche Kunst so befremdet und abgeneigt gegenubergestanden hatten, als wir das in der Gegenwart mit Augen sehen" (163). Nietzsche is against art reduced to "a pleasant sideline" when he writes, "Vielleicht aber wird es fuer eben dieselben ueberhaupt anstoessig sein, ein aesthetische Problem so Ernst genommen zu sehn, falls sie naemlich in der Kunst nicht mehr als ein lustige Nebenbei, als ein auch wohl zu missendes Schellengklinkel zum Ernst des Daseins zu erkennen imstande sind: als ob niemand wusste, was es bei dieser Gegenuberstellung mit einem solchen Ernste des Daseins auf sich habe" (p. 16). Nietzsche asserts that science needs art when he writes, "Wenn er hier zu seinem Schrecken sieht, wie die Logik sich an diesen Grenzen um sich selbst ringlet und endlich sich in den Schwanz beisst- da bricht die neue Form der Erkenntnis durch, die tragische Erkenntnis, die, um nur ertragen zu werden, als Schutz und Heilmittel die Kunst braucht" (p. 130). Since Socrates for Nietzsche represents science the ideal of an artistic science is embodied in a music practicing Socrates.

criteria of scientific method, and exploration. Even medicine should be concerned as a medical art.[43]

Time is precious, and when one is a physician as Maimonides wrote to Ibn Tibbon who inquired about how to translate *The Guide for the Perplexed* (מורה נבוכים) from Arabic *dalālatul ḥā'irīn* דלאלה דלאלה אלחאירין into Hebrew, the Great Philosopher-Talmudist-Physician could only meet on Shabbos between *musaf and minchah* because his week day duties as a physician to the Sultan's court and the Jewish patients in the Jewish quarter was so less "leisurely" than what he knew as a someone fortunate to sit and learn his first 40 years of his life while his brother Rabbi David Maimon (ztsl), in the precious gems business, like Zevulun supporting Yisachar, supported the Great Eagle *(Nesher HaGadol)* to learn that led to the writings of the *Sefer ha-higayon, MT, perush al hamishnah,* and numerous medical texts. Dr. Levy did not have much leisure before retirement due to his devotion 150% to his patients health. Dr. Levy's devotion to the preservation of life and sanctity of life for each patient left little time for leisure. The physicians guide is an imperative to heal for all life is sacred and inviolate. Dr. Levy's example as a physician shows the affirmation of the holy nature of being a physician for man's body and life are not a man's to give away and every effort should be made to reduce pain and increase longevity and quality of life which God gives, for man's life is not his alone, but the property of the God who gives life and happiness.

---

[43] Barzel, Uriel S., "The Art of Cure" : a medical text by Maimonides, Moses Maimonides (1993) 59-63

Dr Levy will be the first to tell you that what he has accomplished is so modest. We may recall Newton's modesty when upon discovering the mathematical formula for gravity, Newton proclaimed that he had discovered a drop of wisdom in the sea of G-d's infinite waters of wisdom. Dr. Levy recognized that the essays in this book are not even the tip of an iceberg, a tincture of significance compared to great medical giants like Albert Schweitzer whose example was one of ethical praxis. Schweitzer is more than a hero of Dr. Levy's for as an inspiration Schweitzer devoted his time to helping underserved populations in the area of public health.[44] Martin Buber's relationship with Schweitzer further proves fascinating and well worth looking into.[45]

Further the intellectual-cognitive giants like Maimonides,[46] *mimosh limoshe likam kimoshe*, puts anyone's own research in perspective as the Rambam wrote seminal ground breaking works in many areas[47] such as Philosophy, Jewish Law, Music and Medicine that continue to make an

---

[44] Paget, James Carleton, Albert Schweitzer and the Jews, Harvard Theological Review 107,3 (2014) 363-398

[45] Stiehm, Lothar, Martin Buber und Albert Schweitzer : Geben, Nehmen, Miteinander 1901-1965, Den Menschen zugewandt leben (1999) 97-116; Vermes, Pamela, The Buber-Schweitzer correspondence., Journal of Jewish Studies 37,2 (1986) 228-245, Spear, Otto, In the view of research - Schweitzer and Buber on the will of Jesus and the idea of the Kingdom of God, Universitas 22,3 (1980) 227-231.

[46] See Collins, Kenneth E, Maimonides as the "ideal physician" - a role model for modern Jewish medical practice., Korot 18 (2006) 9-24.

[47] Gesundheit, Benjamin, Maimonides (1138-1204) : rabbi, physician and philosopher, IMAJ 7,9 (2005) 547-553.

important impact until today.[48] Rambam's legacy is astounding and rare.[49] Rambam's recommendations for people suffering from asthma[50] are as relevant[51] today as in the medieval ages.[52] Even in Dr Levy's field Rambam's analysis of evaluating urine is still relevant today for modern neprhology.[53] Rambam was a physician whose medical way of seeing things even influenced his halakhic decisions.[54]

Dr. Levy's explorations have taken him to libraries, archives, and even the marsh lands of the Maryland eastern shore to explore the wild growing mallow plant described by Homer as good for curing sword wounds. Also his explorations in medical history have taken him into the inner city projects around Hopkins Hospital to document via

[48]   Berner, Herbert, MAIMONIDES—PHYSICIAN, ASTRONOMER, PHILOSOPHER, TALMUDIST, JAMA 1955;157(18):1637. doi:10.1001/jama.1955.02950350051026

[49] Meyerhof, Max, Las obras médicas de Maimónides, Maimónides - médico (2005) 37-76

[50] Shakour, Adel, Relative clauses in Hebrew translation of Maimonides' "Treatise on Asthma.", Hebrew Studies 55 (2014) 117-127

[51] Goodhill, Victor, Maimonides : medical relevance, 1985, Sobre la vida y obra de Maimónides (1991) 273-278.

[52] Moral García, Antonio del, La materia médica en la obra de Maimónides : breve comentario al tratado "Sarh asma'al-'uggar" (Explicación de los nombres de las drogas), obre la vida y obra de Maimónides (1991) 209-217.

[53] Rosner, Fred, Moses Maimonides' aphorisms regarding analysis of urine., Annals of Internal Medicine 71,1 (1969) 217-220

[54] Halperin, Mordecha, Parturition : the medical background of some halakhic Maimonidean rulings, BDD 2 (1996) 41-49

photography the old house where many a old time physician's hero, the great Sir William Osler, lived and resided for much of his life. So too Dr. Levy sought out the library of Osler in Canada's library of the University of Montreal and was truly awed by how great a book collector was Osler. Osler the bibliophile, who collected every edition of the Latin text of *Religio Medici* made medicine and being a physician into a kind of religion. Sir William Osler, a legend to many Hopkins graduates, was a rare soul, scientific pioneer, and helped develop a great organization of Hopkins medical schools. Many afternoons have been spent in the Hopkins Welch Library where the hypnotic hush of the silent stacks have a lure of a sacred space of holy hush that attracts Dr. Levy for its peaceful environment.

Yet the search for knowledge is not static and has motivated Dr. Levy to trek thru snow, ice, and rain to the Hopkins Homewood campus to consult the microfiche and microfilm collections from the Vatican archives, with regards to research of old Latin and Spanish texts from 15th & 16th Spanish explorers, who brought back to Spain medicinal plants, and medicines from "the New World." Part of the excitement of pursuing the truth, wherever it may lead one, and to interact with the various diverse and fascinating persons one meets along the way, is a drive for the process and quest for greater understanding. In the course of Dr. Levy's research he has met scholars, artists, chemists, eccentric scholarly librarians, to literary critics and the whole gamut of humanity. This makes Dr. Levy's research a part of the inter-human and a form of team work.

Dr. Levy recalls many wonderful vital discussions about his research with academic scholars of the history of science at Hopkins such as Oswei Temkin Professor of History of Medicine, and Lawrence M. Principe, Professor of History of Science at JHU.

In Dr. Levy's work one finds a respect for the Humanities to make one's research more sensitive to all artistic disciplines. Dr Levy is familiar with medical metaphors in great works of world literature such as *Death in Venice (Der Tod in Venedig) The Magic Mountain (Die Zauberberg), The Death of Ivan Ilyovitch (Смертъ Ивана Ильича)*. Even while being a busy physician with many duties and responsibilities Dr. Levy set aside time to take his son to attend Dr. Uvrehei' & Professor Richard Macksey's seminars at Hopkins on Literature, Music, and Medicine that spanned the gamut from antiquity to present day film studies. Refreshing breadth, that did not skimp on depth of substance, in an age of narrow specialization conditioned by the post-modern technological revolution, animated these lectures and affirmed the need for caring and well rounded physicians as Renaissnance persons with a wide gamut of multifaced and broad interests.

Dr. Levy has conveyed to me and others the gratitude and excitement of meeting in the course of his research, the brilliant Professor of Chemistry, Dr. Principe of Hopkins, who wrote his dissertation on Robert Boyle and Alchemy (alchemy and chemistry being allied for many millennia in the history of science), and who offered much expert advice, leads, and vast knowledge of the field that he was so graciously willing to share with Dr Levy in this area. Further Dr Levy speaks with great enthusiasm and excitement when discovering that the art department of Hopkins has a special section devoted to the representation in pen, ink, pastel, and now computer imaging and 3D printing of scientific specimens, that proved helpful for his wish to include a picture of the 16th century discovery of the wood—*lignum nephriticum,* in one of his power points. This *lignum nephriticum* was the origin of scientific understanding of not only fluorescents, the later understanding of the properties of acids-bases-salts, but was also considered at the time of its discovery as a possible remedy of the times for kidney problems.

Ergo in the quest for knowledge one never knows where one's journey will lead on to, and where one will end up, either in the halls of professors, the labs of chemists, the libraries and archives of JHU (research of various papers), NYU (research on Homer Smith), or Montreal University (research on Osler) or the marshlands of the eastern shore collecting therapeutic specimens of marsh-mallow for treating wounds. As Robert Frost writes in his poem, "*Swinger of Birch Trees*" about a child who grows up in a rural area of Vermont, far away from any stores, but must innovate and create his own areas of discovery, "surely one could be worse than a swinger of birches." Dr Levy became his own teacher, learning on his own in retirement, motivated by an unquenchable thirst for further knowledge and intellectual adventure. As John Donne knows, "no man is an island," and life is a journey, that is best lived amongst true friends who share the quest for the life of the mind in pursuit of knowledge (*episteme*). Thus the journeys required for writing the following essays in the history of medicine, are offered in intellectual friendship to make a positive contribution. However perhaps more importantly they represent a noble virtuous soul who seeks intellectual work as the highest form of happiness in retirement.[55]

The Osler Society allows Dr Levy to present power point presentations of some of the papers that appear in this collection. This group of historians of medicine and science are not only interested in Osler, although a great number of important biographies have appeared on this seminal luminary in the history of medicine (see Charles S. Bryan's *Osler: Inspirations from a Great Physician*) but form a scholarly group of kindred souls interested in the development of science in general and questions such as what makes for scientific discovery and paradigm shifts. More works on Hopkins greats are appearing such as Michael Bliss' *Harvey Cushing: A Life in Surgery* etc. and the Osler Society continues to toil on behalf of increasing knowledge of the history and development of medicine.

It is not just a matter of Dr. Levy trying to keep his mind active in retirement from which these essays grew, but, a sense of new discoveries ever fresh, like vistas opening up on continuing mental sunrises of understanding. To store up an archival record as Baruch ben Nariah did for Yeremahu, "a message in a bottle", these essays represent also an effort by Dr. Levy to leave a presence of his devotion to the life of the mind.

---

[55] Hava Tirosh-Samuelson, *Happiness in Premodern Judaism: Virtue, Knowledge and Well Being* HUC Monograph #29, 2003.

When Stephen Gould was asked what NASA should put in a spacecraft launched into space for other life forms, as messages in a bottle, Gould recommended the space craft include Bach Cantatas, a copy of the Bible, and Newton's *Principia*. So too these essays are a message in a bottle of Dr Levy's intellectual work. They celebrate in most idealistic form a wish to write one's own resurrection symphony, as Mozart did as dramatically portrayed in the film, *Amadeus*, as noted in volume One on *Music and Medicine*. If all humans desire to ultimately be caught up in eternity, perpetual peace, then real lasting achievement rests not on fame, prestige, or anything physically pleasurable, but if one has experienced by thinking true thoughts, true for all peoples at all times, regardless of cultural and geographical differences, entering into what is not finite, what is true, good, and beautiful by nature of the life of the mind as quest and journey for knowledge as a virtue (arête). It is not the end or output that is important. It is this process of quest and journey devoted to the search that makes a difference when infused with love of knowledge and a wish to share it with others.

Academically researchers make a positive contribution to the content of knowledge, and move the academic discussion along adding illuminating insights, that hopefully benefit the human community in intellectual understanding, informed by an ethical culture. Dr Levy's interest in harmonizing the Humanities with science and medicine is an effort at endearing an ethical culture of science.[56] Derrida's *Archive Fever in* name speaks to the desire for being a part of something greater than the limits of "the solipsism of the self", and perhaps it is only when we serve others, and their needs with ethical commitment, that we leave our good deeds to future generations and future memory, in an attempt to share and benefit others. By publishing these essays, which Dr Levy was reluctant to due out of his sense of perfectionism and modesty, archival memory is served by preserving not so much the end product of these essays, but a trace of the noble quest that led to their writing. Works of history, art, and philosophy enter.... ideally into a testimony that life has meaning and can be redeemed by intellectual research and should partake of the perpetual peace of the eternality that is *truth/aletheia/veritas/wahrheit/ emes*. Like *Yakov Avinu* Dr. Levy is a man of truth (*notain emet li-Yakov*) He recognizes that by the nature of histories warp and weft every expression in the Humanities and science is an expression of the spirit of its time. Yet what these essays express is something very old and noble. It is an affirmation of the importance of intellectual pursuit, journey, and quest without any alterieur motives, but solely as a good unto itself for, this quest affirms man's being made *BiTzelem Elokim* by affirming the existence of the active intellect and its being guided by an ethical vision, and sharing that vision with others.

Dizzying velocities of change due to the technological revolution characterized by Jean

---

[56] See Lieber, Elinor, Maimonides the medical humanist, Maimonidean Studies 4 (2000) 39-60

Lyotard as *The Post-Modern Condition*,[57] have made the multifaceted well rounded Renaissance man[58] a rare example indeed, and these essays celebrate the need for physicians not to become so myopic in their gaze as to forget the larger picture, to mistake the forest for the trees. The Renaissance Man must know both science and the Humanities which he makes to work in tandem. Thus while Arthur Cohen[59] had many wide interests it is not clear whether he was grounded in science although his book, *The Tremendum*, deserves to be read over and over again. Perhaps we may think of the Renaissance man *avant la lettre* as Rambam's prize student Joseph (Aknin) for whom he wrote Sefer Moreh HaNevukhim, in which in part the Rambam set out to reconcile science and torah[60], as Joseph knew both science and rabbinic texts, that is to say he lived in both Straussian worlds of Athens (Science) and Jerusalem (revealed religion)?

Dr Levy is from a different earlier age when house calls, were made by physicians. This is not to be

---

[57] Lyotard, Jean François, The postmodern condition : a report on knowledge, Minneapolis : University of Minnesota Press, 1984

[58] Berek, Peter, The Jew as Renaissance man, Renaissance Quarterly 51,1 (1998) 128-162

[59] Cole, Diane, Profession: Renaissance man - Arthur A. Cohen, Present Tense 9, 1 (1981) 32-35

[60] http://libguides.tourolib.org/scienceandtorah

confused with Kafka's "Country doctor"[61] who like
many of Kafka's characters yearns to transcend the
bureaucratic Kafquesque nightmare as in *Das*

---

[61] Ein Landarzt.

Ich war in großer Verlegenheit: eine dringende Reise stand mir bevor; ein
Schwerkranker wartete auf mich in einem zehn Meilen entfernten Dorfe; starkes
Schneegestöber füllte den] weiten Raum zwischen mir und ihm; einen Wagen
hatte ich, leicht, großräderig, ganz wie er für unsere Landstraßen taugt; in den
Pelz gepackt, die Instrumententasche in der Hand, stand ich reisefertig schon auf
dem Hofe; aber das Pferd fehlte, das Pferd. Mein eigenes Pferd war in der letzten
Nacht, infolge der Überanstrengung in diesem eisigen Winter, verendet; mein
Dienstmädchen lief jetzt im Dorf umher, um ein Pferd geliehen zu bekommen;
aber es war aussichtslos, ich wußte es, und immer mehr vom Schnee überhäuft,
immer unbeweglicher werdend, stand ich zwecklos da. Am Tor erschien das
Mädchen, allein, schwenkte die Laterne; natürlich, wer leiht jetzt sein Pferd her
zu solcher Fahrt? Ich durchmaß noch einmal den Hof; ich fand keine
Möglichkeit; zerstreut, gequält stieß ich mit dem Fuß an die brüchige Tür des
schon seit Jahren unbenützten Schweinestalles. Sie öffnete sich und klappte in
den Angeln auf und zu. Wärme und Geruch wie von Pferden kam hervor. Eine
trübe Stallaterne schwankte drin an einem Seil. Ein Mann, zusammengekauert in
dem niedrigen Verschlag, zeigte sein offenes blauäugiges Gesicht. »Soll ich
anspannen?« fragte er, auf allen Vieren hervorkriechend. Ich wußte nichts zu
sagen und beugte mich nur, um zu sehen, was es noch in dem Stalle gab. Das
Dienstmädchen stand neben mir. »Man weiß nicht, was für Dinge man im
eigenen Hause vorrätig hat, sagte es, und wir beide lachten. »Hollah, Bruder,
hollah, Schwester rief der Pferdeknecht, und zwei Pferde, mächtige flankenstarke
Tiere schoben sich hintereinander, die Beine eng am Leib, die wohlgeformten
Köpfe wie Kamele senkend, nur durch die Kraft der Wendungen ihres Rumpfes
aus dem Türloch, das sie restlos ausfüllten. Aber gleich standen sie aufrecht,
hochbeinig, mit dicht ausdampfendem Körper. »Hilf ihm,« sagte ich, und das
willige Mädchen eilte, dem Knecht das Geschirr des Wagens zu reichen. Doch
kaum war es bei ihm, umfaßt es der Knecht und schlägt sein Gesicht an ihres
……Der Arzt ist Euch ins Bett gelegt!«

Niemals komme ich so nach Hause; meine blühende Praxis ist verloren; ein
Nachfolger bestiehlt mich, aber ohne Nutzen, denn er kann mich nicht ersetzen;
in meinem Hause wütet der ekle Pferdeknecht; Rosa ist sein Opfer; ich will es
nicht ausdenken. Nackt, dem Froste dieses unglückseligsten Zeitalters[33]
ausgesetzt, mit irdischem Wagen, unirdischen Pferden, treibe ich mich alter
Mann umher. Mein Pelz hängt hinten am Wagen, ich kann ihn aber nicht
erreichen, und keiner aus dem beweglichen Gesindel der Patienten rührt den
Finger. Betrogen! Betrogen! Einmal dem Fehlläuten der Nachtglocke gefolgt – es
ist niemals gutzumachen.

Schloos[62], and *Vor Dem Gesetz*, and other stories. Kafka's stories yearn for a demonstration of careingness that goes into attending to the well being of the patient, for whom the physician's oath swears to do no damages, to relieve pain, and to extend and enhance the quality and longevity of life, etc. Kafka understood that the *house call of a country doctor* makes the doctor into a healer devoted to humanity and its benefit and not just an expert cold objective scientist who might be replaced by a robot. Rather being a healer, means caring for one's patients and affirming the sanctification of life and imperative to heal all

---

[62] Walter Benjamin, Illuminations, " (New York: Schocken Books), p. 112. Kafka provides us with an intimate detail of bureaucracies inefficiencies. In chapter five of The Castle, the mayor gives an intricate scenario of K's lost file. K. tells the major that his story is amusing because it gives "an insight into the ludicrous bungling that in certain circumstances may decide the life of a human being." Olga sums up the nature of bureaucracy when she says, "One can never find out exactly what is happening, or a long time afterwards." Often the bureaucracy makes mistakes as in the case when K. is sent a letter praising him for work he has not done. The maze of bureaucracy separates K. from the castle. Kafka reveals the dark side of bureaucracy that can cause the individual to feel like a nonentity. In chapter 20 of the Castle, the narrator recounts how the chambermaids who wait on the secretaries feel "lost and forgotten" as if they were working down in a mine. K. is a supplicant "down below" who aspires to enter the Castle "up above" but is denied access by the bureaucracy, accounting for what Thomas Mann called the "humanly unassailable transcendent." Thomas Mann, Homage to Franz Kafka (New York: Knopf, 1984).

humanity. Thus Kafka's parable *Vor Dem Gesetz*[63] can be viewed as describing those gatekeepers of different ranks, who due to merit gained in *olam ha-zeh* are set up to provide access to the next palace chamber in the labyrinth of the hierarchical structure of the seven heavens (hechalot), i.e. gatekeepers of various sorts—gatekeepers as shaluchim of health, gate keepers of knowledge, gate keepers of ethical sanctification, gatekeepers of goodness, etc who serve as door keepers in the

---

[63] Kafka writes, "Vor dem Gesetz steht ein Turhuter. Zu diesem Turhuter kommt ein Mann vom Lande und bittet um Eintritt in das Gesetz. Aber der Turhuter sagt, dass er ihm jetzt den Eintritt nicht gewahren konne. Der Mann uberlegt und fragt dann, ob er also spatter werde eintreten durfen. `Es ist moeglich, sagt der Turhuter, jetzt aber nicht. Da das Tor zum Gesetz offensteht wie immer und der Turhuter beiseite tritt, buckt sich der Mann, um durch das Tor in das Innere zu sehen. Als der Turhuter das merkt, lacht er und sagt: `Wenn es dich so lockt, versuche es doch trotz meines Verbotes hineinzugehen. Merke aber: Ich bin machtig. Und ich bin nur der unterste Turhuter. Von Saal zu Saal stehen aber Turhuter, einer machtiger als der andere. Schon den Anblick des dritten kann nicht einmal ich mehr ertragen.' Solche Schwierigkeiten hat der Mann vom Lande nicht erwartet; das Gesetz soll doch jedem und immer zuganglich sein, denkt er, aber als er jetzt den Turhuter in seinem Pelzmantel genauer ansieht, seine grosse Spitznase, den langen, dunnen, schwarzen tatarischen Bart, entschliesst er sich, doch lieber zu warten, bis er die Erlaubnis zum Eintritt bekommt. Der Turhuter gibt ihm einen Schemel und lasst ihn seitwarts von der Tur sich niedersetzen. Dort sitzt er Tage und Jahre. Er macht viele Versuche, eingelassen zu werden, und ermudet den Turhuter durch seine Bitten. Der Turhuter stellt ofters kleine Verhore mit ihm an, fragt ihn uber seine Heimat aus und nach vielem anderen, es sind aber teilnahmslose Fragen, wie sie grosse Herren stellen, und zum Schlusse sagt er ihm immer wieder, dass er ihn noch nicht einlassen konne.

form of the Turhuter.[64] While Kafka's work depicts the inhuman side of bureaucracy, and speaks to an essential need for the human side of the human condition to triumph over the impersonal machine like bureaucratic process, Dr Levy's role in medicine always never lost sight of the human being behind the patient rather than a bureaucratic statistic. Today medicine has become more bureaucratic and more technical. The fusion of bureaucracy and technology or technocracy risks effacing the human side of the physician as a practitioner devoted to the benefit of the health of their patients. Technology is a two edged sword

---

[64] Kafka writes, "Vor dem Gesetz steht ein Turhuter. Zu diesem Turhuter kommt ein Mann vom Lande und bittet um Eintritt in das Gesetz. Aber der Turhuter sagt, dass er ihm jetzt den Eintritt nicht gewahren konne. Der Mann uberlegt und fragt dann, ob er also spatter werde eintreten durfen. `Es ist moeglich, sagt der Turhuter, jetzt aber nicht. Da das Tor zum Gesetz offensteht wie immer und der Turhuter beiseite tritt, buckt sich der Mann, um durch das Tor in das Innere zu sehen. Als der Turhuter das merkt, lacht er und sagt: `Wenn es dich so lockt, versuche es doch trotz meines Verbotes hineinzugehen. Merke aber: Ich bin machtig. Und ich bin nur der unterste Turhuter. Von Saal zu Saal stehen aber Turhuter, einer machtiger als der andere. Schon den Anblick des dritten kann nicht einmal ich mehr ertragen.' Solche Schwierigkeiten hat der Mann vom Lande nicht erwartet; das Gesetz soll doch jedem und immer zuganglich sein, denkt er, aber als er jetzt den Turhuter in seinem Pelzmantel genauer ansieht, seine grosse Spitznase, den langen, dunnen, schwarzen tatarischen Bart, entschliesst er sich, doch lieber zu warten, bis er die Erlaubnis zum Eintritt bekommt. Der Turhuter gibt ihm einen Schemel und lasst ihn seitwarts von der Tur sich niedersetzen. Dort sitzt er Tage und Jahre. Er macht viele Versuche, eingelassen zu werden, und ermudet den Turhuter durch seine Bitten. Der Turhuter stellt ofters kleine Verhore mit ihm an, fragt ihn uber seine Heimat aus und nach vielem anderen, es sind aber teilnahmslose Fragen, wie sie grosse Herren stellen, und zum Schlusse sagt er ihm immer wieder, dass er ihn noch nicht einlassen konne. See Jacques Derrida, "Devant la Loi," in Kafka and the Contemporary Critical Performance (Bloomington and Indianapolis: Indiana Univeristy Press, 1987), pp. 128-150. When Morgan notes that Scholem treats Kafka as a neo-Kabbalist, giving new readings of revelation" (p. 67) we cannot help asking if Scholem would view the gatekeeper of "Vor Dem Gesetz" as analogous to mystical descriptions of various angels as archons of differing rank, who guard the heavenly halls of the seven heavens?

which can save life and at the same time lead to its devolution.[65]

In some way the essays in this volume speak to the importance not only of intellectual discovery that arose from their research, but reconnecting the fragmented overly technocratic world with its human side, a side that should be able to empathize with others, and share with others, and relate to others in some vision of medicine as an ethical culture.

Doctoring has come a long way since Shakespeare's father-in-law the apothecary. It is one thing to research as Dr Levy has into uncovering the actual

---

[65] See Blog post at https://tclibraryblog.wordpress.com/2018/01/24/libraries-archives-and-technology-in-post-modern-times/ There we read, "On one hand, biotechnology has promoted the longevity and quality of life. For example, organ transplants and pain elimination enhance the value provided by the medical profession. Soon, advances in stem cell research and cloning may allow engineered biological enhancements (such as eye implants to enable night vision) and end diseases through reverse genetic engineering. Thus, we understand Friedrich Hölderlin's poetic verse in "Patmos": "Where the danger is, there is the saving power too." Of course, these new scientific advances raise many important ethical and moral questions in the rapid advance of biotechnology. See, for instance, our LibGuides on: Humanistic Medicine, Jewish Ethics, Jews in Medicine, Internet and Online Ethics, and Philosophy of Science. Yet, technology may be a two-edged sword. Technology exploited by sinister elements for nefarious ends could lead to nuclear Armageddon if the one-dimensional Marcusian Buberian I-IT relationship triumphs above all. What Nietzsche described as the "will to power" and Heidegger refers to as the essence of technology being Control (Gestell) means we must look thoughtfully and critically into this "two-edged sword" which has the power for both immense good and immense evil. As archivists traditionally seek to preserve, conserve and leave traces of civilization and the afterlife of events, the question becomes how that is done in an age when technological footprints are in constant flux and knowledge is no longer seen as static, but constantly evolving in different formats. What is being done by archivists today to preserve traces of our now "current- past" (intentional oxymoron) civilization? Media archivist Wolfgang Ernst (see Digital Memory) pioneers the field of media archaeology (archivology) which uncovers and excavates not the role of specific technologies, but infrastructures that structure what is possible for humans to do and achieve in potential for arriving at media historical knowledge, and mechanisms in shaping culture and memory in digital culture. Archives are no longer just a static body of knowledge, but rather an ever-changing interactive fluid dynamic outside of human control. The constantly-changing nature of the contents of the digital archive point to a James Joycean simulacrum, Kafkaesque reality (see "Before the Law" in The Trial) of ambiguity & flux, and a Beckett-like anticlimactic Waiting for Godot post-modern condition. Derrida (in Archive Fever) notes that this post-modern condition risks the slippery slope of being unable to tell the difference between intelligence from artificial intelligence, historical artifact, real time in the philosophical understanding, and consciousness. Not only is culture (see Neil Postman) at stake, but thinking itself, upon which de Tocqueville says democracy exists of, falls. Technology also leads to many problems. One problem is addiction to its use. More is needed than just partial solutions like 'Camp Grounded', 'Digital Detox,' and the Age of Techno-Anxiety to disconnect only temporarily from a menacing threat that risks denuding the human being in the image of G-d, and the place for the sacred (Mander, 1992). Unplugging temporarily will not save us, according to Jurgenson, who argues that virtual reality risks replacing understanding of the real reality. In the Absence of the Sacred: The Failure of Technology discusses a frenetic age of technocracy (fusion of bureaucracy and technology) that threatens to reduce all causality, including escalating of military confrontations with weapons of mass destruction, "to a reporting" (see The Question Concerning Technology) that is susceptible to the "technological glitch", not to mention "tampered technologically generated data", hacking, data breaches, identity theft, etc, eliminating thinking itself by computing. Technology has also led to a 1984-type Orwellian slouching described, in part, by Bernard Harcourt. We live in an age where network service providers, search engines, and social media monitor our every digital action, potentially eradicating freedoms, privacy, and thought itself. Another problem is that students sometimes falsely believe that with the click of a mouse their assignment is easily done, when in reality the hard work of reading critically, analyzing, thinking, and creatively presenting a case has not begun. Accordingly, the effort is the reward! What is the place of libraries and archives in this Borgean labyrinthian (see Borges' short story, The Library of Babel) reality that dare not be trumped by virtual reality? It is not just fact-checking and knowing how to access "information" (see Jean-Francois Lyotard, The Postmodern Condition: A Report on Knowledge), it is the resistance to the eradication of true thinking that penetrates to the depths and roots of problems, and offers not a superficial panacea to its rectification but a final solution to guarding the freedoms, dignity, and transcendence of the life of the mind, and search for intellectual, moral, and spiritual virtue. The danger grows as we have evolved at risk from the school of Protagoras that mistakenly held man is the measure of all things to a worse state where machines have dangerously become the measure of all things."

medicines in the Shakespearean oeuvre where the Bard in *Hamlet* alludes to a poison for Claudius' ear, and in *Romeo and Juliet* the star crossed lovers, take a sleeping potion, the substance of which has been classified in the scatter of the literature, and quite another more important accomplishment for a man of science to feel the emotional and vibrant nature of the Shakespearean depiction of the gamut of the emotions and diversity of characters representing the human condition. The verse in the Bard's play "what says the physician to my water?...."

Uroscopy is mentioned in the Shakespearean canon. Macbeth's request to the "doctor of physic" to "cast / The water of my land, find her disease / And purge it to a sound and pristine health" (5.3.52–54). Less momentously, let us recall Falstaff's first line in *2 Henry IV*, "*what says the doctor to my water?*" (1.2.1). In moments of the greatest enormity, Shakespeare cites uroscopy as a device for the determination of pathology whether that be on the scale of an entire country or the self-inflicted waning of the fat Fastaffian comic knight.

Uroscopy had various practical advantages. It was, unlike hematoscopy, nonintrusive. It was cheap and since, like Falstaff's, the sample was often carried to the uroscopist, it required neither a home-visit (more expensive) nor the movement of the possibly nonambulant patient. In fact, the profession of urine courier emerged at this time— the so-called "piss messenger." Furthermore, since the patient was not required to be present, a degree of anonymity could be maintained, which was particularly welcome in cases where uroscopy was used to determine whether or not a woman was pregnant. According to one anonymous source of 1599, if an inspection of the urine reflected the face of the uroscopist, this was a sure sign of pregnancy

The ubiquity and longevity of this diagnostic method of uroscopy has a long history predating Shakesepare's renaissance England. In antiquity soothsayers engaged in "urine prophecy," or "uromancy" to predict the future and course of things. In the middle ages when the glass flask, known as a matula, was used more, it is noteworthy in shape as a conspicuous visual echoe of paintings of the alchemist at work with a similar type of vessel when engaging in alchemy which as late as the time of Robert Boyle was a hard core science and not considered a magical delusion. Paintings of uroscopists, often set against a background of paraphernalia of the uroscopist's study—globes, charts, copies of learned books on botany, medicine, and anatomy. And the presence of such Faustian objects is conveys to the viewers of these paintings that the healer is by no means an uneducated charlatan but a learned wizard like physician. Despite the erudition and mystification of the uroscopist's profession, the advent of clinical medicine and especially advances in anatomy, put uroscopy of a much more solid epistemological foundations as a modern science and method and empirical research. Urinalysis thus eventually replaced the wizard like methods of uroscopy.

Speaks to a urological knowledge of Renaissance England on uroscopy, but much more of importance, represents the physician as an interpreter of signs in the service of promoting health. As everyone may be likened to a "text" we all would do well to interpret the signs of the texts we meet, and more importantly see each human being as a text yearning to be interpreted.

Much has been written on science in the Renaissance particularly in Italy where Friedenwald, Robert Bonfil, and David Ruderman have documented that greater numbers of Jews were allowed to attend medical schools. Ruderman has also written an excellent book titled, *Jewish thought and scientific discovery in early modern Europe.* Physicians in the future ever becoming technological age are, braced upon the window of which we are seeing the Nietzschean abyss... not hopefully to loose sight of the forest for the trees. Books like Stowe's *Doctoring the South: Southern Physicians and Everyday medicine in the Mid-Nineteenth Century* in part is a book that bares reading to see what medicine for better or worse has left, as it becomes more and more global and international in size and scope, often conscripted by the technological forms it adopted in the name of economic efficiency and innovation. Technology can save lives as with the dialysis machine and kidney transplants. Yet we must not forget *Die Frage ueber der Technologie* of continental philosophy: *Wo die Gefahr ist, wachste das retende auch* (where the danger is there is the saving power too) for technology can save lives as in medicine, but when used by fame-power-seeking Macbethian Machiavelian politicians (Leo Strauss identifies Macavelli as the teacher of evil) devoid of an understanding of the "common good", we dare not let technology lead to nuclear Armageddon, as Einstein feared after World War II in advocating for arms reduction and constraints on production of weapons of mass destruction. Out of *Ahavas Olam, Amor Mundi,* we must resist the dangers technology poses when used by irresponsible politicians, which can lead, when "causality in the news media shrinks to a reporting." When causality shrinks to a reporting the danger of escalation of military confrontations is at risk. Political events and actions can happen more quickly. Causality has shrunken to reporting in the post-modern condition due to velocities of change caused by instant messaging, the internet, email, texting etc. While in the middle ages one must send out a horseman with a letter to relay news, or a pigeon with a note on its foot, in the modern technological era things can happen almost instantaneously. News itself can be crafted by political spin doctors for hire who may wish to set and configure mass opinion amongst the hoi polio for ulterior motives and political agendas. De Toqueville feared that an uneducated public would make disastrous decisions in a democracy such as the U.S. which is not really a democracy as long as the electoral College and gerrymandering operates. Tyrannical demagogues can come to power, and irresponsibly and unqualifiedly make disastrous choices that lead to nuclear Armageddon. Often decision time is eliminated by the technological post-modern condition because those making decisions whether to respond to an alleged invasion by missiles must rely on radar, computer simulation, and algorithms whereby the window to make decisions and choices is relegated to a machine or computer that can map out the chess board consequences more easily than the time a human brain can calculate. The problem is that computers can store mass amounts of data and compute, but they do not have moral or ethical responsibility, unlike this potential in humans. Humanistic science and medicine is a call for an ethical culture and science is one type of culture.

The flip side of technology that we should celebrate as the "saving power' are the miracles of science in the field of medicine for employing technology to extend longevity and quality of lives, as in advance made in kidney transplants.

While the "house call" has been phased out by doctors who may mistakingly view medicine as a profession, and not a calling,[66] that it is not lucrative financially to visit only perhaps one remotely located patient in the middle of an isolated place, perhaps we might recall the altruistic Albert Schweitzer who made a lifelong house call to the tribes of Africa, building the hospital with his own hands, striving to wipe out malaria, and living in a tent most of his whole life, denying himself even a piano or organ, for the music he so loved to play (as the author of a two volume set on Bach and accomplished organist and pianist). Schweitzer as a graduate of Harvard could have had any door open to him, yet chose to live in

---

[66] Clearly in Maimonides Oath medicine is conceived of as an ethical calling: "The eternal providence has appointed me to watch over the life and health of Thy creatures. May the love for my art actuate me at all time; may neither avarice nor miserliness, nor thirst for glory or for a great reputation engage my mind; for the enemies of truth and philanthropy could easily deceive me and make me forgetful of my lofty aim of doing good to Thy children. May I never see in the patient anything but a fellow creature in pain.
Grant me the strength, time and opportunity always to correct what I have acquired, always to extend its domain; for knowledge is immense and the spirit of man can extend indefinitely to enrich itself daily with new requirements. Today he can discover his errors of yesterday and tomorrow he can obtain a new light on what he thinks himself sure of today. Oh, God, Thou has appointed me to watch over the life and death of Thy creatures; here am I ready for my vocation and now I turn unto my calling."

poverty in Africa totally devoted to the medical needs of the local underdeveloped population. Today we need more role models in medicine like Albert Schweitzer. We need more physicians motivated by the healers calling rather than professionalism. Schweitzer's lived example is a refreshing model, whose good deeds resound in the symphony of creation, like the trout in Franz Schubert's musical piece, whose jump from the glacial Alpine lake and slap upon the unpolluted waters, auf die wasser zu Singen, echoes as an "AMEN" in the musical offering gliding upon the waters in a rowboat with his eyes to the starry heavens at night, where the panoply of the myriads of stars, the eyes of angels, beam down to the musician gliding across the lake.

Researchers today stand on the shoulders of giants. In the field of the history of the Jews in medicine one can benefit greatly in knowledge from scholars like Julius Preus (*Biblical and Talmudic Medicine*), Harry Friedenwald (*History of the Jews in Medicine*)[67], David Macht (*The Heart and Blood in the Bible*), Frank Heynick (*Jews and Medicine: An Epic Saga*), J.M. Efron (*Medicine and the German Jews*), Natalia Berger (*Jews and Medicine*), Fred Rosner (most aspects of Jewish medicine), Gad Freudenthal (*Science in the Medieval Hebrew and Arabic Traditions*) etc. Today Dr. Levy also enjoys and finds discovery in the works of many

---

[67] See http://libguides.tourolib.org/jewsmedicine

philosophers of science and historians of medicine.[68]

Halakhah and medicine is also a growing area of research for rabbinic scholars such as Rabbis David Bleich, Basil Herring, Lord Jacobovits (ztsl), Eliot Dorff, Avraham Steinberg, and the editors of an important 2 vols. (2006) set titled *Jewish Medical Ethics 1989-2004*, by the Dr. Falk Schlesinger

---

[68] In the field of the history of medicine and science in general one can learn much from the likes of Thomas Kuhn (*the Structure of Scientific Revolutions*), Peter Bowler & Iwan Rhys Morus (*Making Modern Science)*, William Eamon (Science and the Secrets of Nature), Paolo Rossi (*The Birth of Modern Science*), Willbur Applebaum (*The Scientific Revolution and the Foundations of Modern Science*), Shapin, Steven (*The Scientific Revolution; The Scientific Life; A social history of Truth*), David Lindberg (The Beginnings of Western Science- 2 vols.), John Henry (*The Scientific Revolution and the Origins of Modern Science*), William Newman (*Atoms and Alchemy*), Andras Gedeon (Science and Technology in Medicine), M. L. Jone's (*The Good Life in the Scientific Revolution*), Lisa Jardine (*Ingenious Pursuits: Building the Scientific Revolution*), etc. In the more narrow history of medicine we have witnessed important volumes such as those by Roy Porter (*The Cambridge history of Medicine*), Jacalyn Duffin (*History of Medicine: A scandalously Short Introduction* [the book is only 432 pages!], W.F. Bynum & Anne Hardy & Christopher Lawrence's work: *The Western Medical Tradition: 1800 to 2000*. Currently the project by Cambridge University press is to release a multivolume encyclopedia on the history of science which at the time of this writing have included, (eds. David C. Lindberg & Ronald I. Numbers), vol. 1 *Ancient Science* (ed by Alexander Jones), *Medieval Science*, vol.2 (eds. David C. Lindberg & Lorraine Daston), Early Modern Science, vol 3 (Katherine Park and Lorraine Daston), Eighteenth Century Science, vol. 4 (ed. Roy Porter), The Modern Physical and Mathematical Sciences, vol. 5 (eds. Mary Jo Nye), *The Modern Biological and Earth Sciences*, vol. 6 (eds. Peter Bowler and John Pickstone), *The Modern Social Sciences*, vol. 7 (eds. Theodore M. Porter and Dorothy Ross), *Modern Science in National and International Context*, vol. 8 (David N. Livingstone and Ronald L. Numbers).

Institute for medical-halahkic research i.e. Drs. Mordecai Halperin, David Fink, and Shimon Glick.[69] These Halakhicists are interested in the relationship also of science and torah.[70]

Today more than ever medicine needs to hear the *moral voice of consciousness*, in a post-modern age that has witnessed the consequences of Machiavellian politics, which Leo Strauss predicted, would lead to Nazi Eugenics bankrupt of any moral and ethical substance, whereby Jewish concentration inmates became lab rats for evil scientists sadistic experiments who inflicted great torture and suffering on innocent prisoners slated for annihilation. How medicine and science hit bottom, is just damning when human beings were viewed as so much "stuff" (*menschen stuffen*) to be used cruelly in the process of "*sonderbehandlung*" (a euphemism for special treatment).

---

[69] Works like the *Tzits Eliezer*, and classical Talmudim, codes (Tur, MT, Shulchan Arukh), and the vast Responsa texts of sheolot ve-teshuvot, analogize apparently new medical realities like IVF, heart-lung machines, cloning, and stem cell research to classic rabbinic case law. Ergo the question of whether to ask the wood chopper to stop chopping wood, or to refrain from administering salt to the tongue of a goses (terminally ill patient) is analogized to the question if when, if ever can one ethically be permitted to discontinue life support. Criteria of death: heartbeat (circulation), breath fogging a mirror (respiration), or brain activity is analogized from classic case law to modern situations. Rabbi Yitzak Breitowitz has written an essential moral and ethical critique of the terrible injustice done to Terry Schiavo, and the dangerous precedent this makes, for future medical decisions, when medicine is interfered with by the most vulgar politcal utilitarian self serving means., The field of medical halakhah is immense and constantly growing, as the oral law, continues to deal with post-modern medicine.

[70] See http://libguides.tourolib.org/scienceandtorah

An ideal researcher will see the forest for the trees, the big sublime picture {which is not a picture at all that can be framed by a border-limit}, for The transcendent Creator dare not be put in a box, for when one does that they relegate G-d to a system....when in fact not being finite, a circle whose circumference is infinite, a sublime power that makes for salvation, defies any attempt to control or manipulate that which is omnipotent]. When the Nazi Selection officers would usurp, the place of G-d as if on Yom Kippur in deciding "who should live"[71] (to the right) and who should die (to the left) then humanity touched moral bankruptcy of the bottom.[72] The need for an ethical culture of science and medicine is thus all the more pressing.

---

[71] Cynthia Ozick's short story *"the shawl "* makes much dramatic effect of this to the right for hard work and to the left to be gassed as does the William Styron's novel *Sophie's Choice*. Also see Tadeusz Borowski's *This Way for the Gas, Ladies and Gentlemen*. In some sense (S)Election becomes Election.

[72] Wetzell, Richard F, Eugenics, racial science, and Nazi biopolitics : was there a Genesis of the "final solution" from the spirit of science?, Beyond the Racial State (2017) 147-175; Allison, Kirk C., Eugenics, race hygiene, and the Holocaust : antecedents and consolidations., The Routledge History of the Holocaust (2011) 45-58; Glad, John, Eugenics and the Holocaust, 1927-1939., Mankind Quarterly 48,4 (2008) 444-483; Czech, Herwig, From welfare to selection : Vienna's public health office and the implementation of racial hygiene policies under the Nazi regime., Blood and Homeland" (2007) 317-333; Weindling, Paul, Central Europe confronts German racial hygiene : Friedrich Hertz, Hugo Iltis and Ignaz Zollschan as critics of racial hygiene., "Blood and Homeland" (2007) 263-280; Pollefeyt, Didier, The significance of Nazi eugenics for medical ethics today, Humanity at the Limit (2000) 250-256; Koonz, Claudia, Genocide and eugenics : the language of power, Lessons and Legacies (1991) 155-177; Dietrich, Donald J., catholic resistance to biological and racist eugenics in the Third Reich, Germans against Nazism (1990) 137-155.

When Prometheus first took fire from the gods, he thereupon offered the Western world the likes of scientific inquiry the myth has it. Likewise it was that philosophic genius, Plato's Socrates, who went around asking the question, "what is X..... (*ti ti esti*) which in essence allowed Nietzsche to view Socrates as the embodiment of the scientific impulse, that Nietzsche may have mistakenly attributed to a cyclops narrowness of myopic vision that had become monstrous in the modern world that he identified in crisis. Leo Strauss defends the Platonic Socrates before its Nietzschean critique in *Die Geburde Der Tragedie*.[73] Rather science when practiced with an understanding to the long view and big picture, which is not a picture with a frame/limit/boundry/border. For true medical practice in that it embodies the ethical world of praxis, is to do good and serve a beneficent power that makes for even redemption. Life is so precious, that the rabbis see the principle of *pekuah nefesh*, mandating in some cases suspending the laws of shabbos, i.e. "let him violate one shabbos so that the patient may observe many shabbatot....(*Yoma* 85b) Or "if we do brit *milah on shabbos*, then kal wa-homer, *minoris ad majoris*, we would do *pekuah nefesh* to save all limbs of the human being, because extending longevity and quality of life can never have a price tag. The Talmud reasons the principle of *pikuah nefesh* from the verse *vachai bahem*, "you shall live by them" (*Vayikra* 18:5). Life is of infinite worth as the Rabbis knew when they likened every human being to "a world" unto themselves.

---

[73] http://libguides.tourolib.org/ld.php?content_id=34501950

Nietzsche urged that there come into being a musical practicing Socrates that could combine the objective critical analysis, and application of objective criteria to solve problems, with the art that is present in disciplines like Music. Thus the Apollonian (god of Music and medicine) would counter the mindless Dionysian (hedonistic wine drinking unbridled wildness that makes for forgetfulness and worse lack of Care-Sorge of the nihilism the West has entered and Nietzsche perceived with great trepidation). While the scientist calls for a strong cup of coffee to wake us up from our slumbers of ignorance, it is Dioynesius who intoxicates his tempted hedonists with the wine of forgetfulness. Science is a wake up call, as the Rambam likens the blasts of the shofar on *Yamim Noraim*, to see reality as it is- the *ding an sich,* and for that science is still allied with the philosophical discipline of epistemology, that asks questions such as: *What is knowledge?, what are the limits of scientific knowledge?, How i.e. by what methods, can we know anything at all?, and by what scientific discipline?* As late as the 18th Century Newton still received a doctorate in philosophy, for as late as the 1700s to do philosophy one must have the prerequisites to know science and its methods.

Newton (1642-1727) was a polymath and autodidactic, and his *Principia* a classic in the field of science. With Archimedes who described "the Eureka Moment" when he mathematically mapped the numeric formula for the displacement of volume, Newton's Eureka moments were not just limited to mapping the mathematical equation for gravity sublunar. Galileo (1564-1642: Astronomer, physicist, engineer, philosopher, mathematician) as a martyr for the truth, loved the truth more than his own physical safety, and unlike Descartes who with caution withheld his mathematical findings that the earth revolves around the sun, Galileo released into the public domain, and thus affirmed his understanding of truth against all the for over 2 millennia domination of the Aristotelian cosmology upon which the church had an invested interest in its commitment to the likes of St. Thomas Aquinas, an Aristotelian who read Maimonide's Guide in a Latin translation, *Doctor Perplexus*. Bertolt Brecht makes this Galilean courage and commitment to "truth" as Galileo understood it post Kepler (1571-1630) and Copernicus (1473-1543), so ennobling that indeed following in the footsteps of Socrates, another martyr of philosophy suffered due to being caught in the web of politics.

When one returns to that man, "more sinned against than sinning" (not as Shakespeare employs that phrase in King Lear III, scene 2 57-60), the man who was put to death to drink the hemlock. Socraties in *the Crito*, chose not to flee, as Aristotle did to Asia Minor, when political forces sought to kill him, we see confirmation of Leo Strauss' thesis of the danger of truth to the multitudes of the many, the *olam* is a *golem*... Socrates as a philosopher and scientist who did no one any real harm, but was condemned as "a sophist" and corrupting the youth without just cause. Because the Athenian state politicians put a just man to death, namely Plato's Socrates, we must wonder why the last words of that scientific philosopher were that he owes a rooster to Aeschlepius the god of healing, perhaps because Socrates as a midwife of ideas, helping give birth of the ideas of others to discover in his Socratic method with the employment of much Socratic irony, some better understanding of the truth, on the road to more and more knowledge, a desire without an end of desire, a desire which Spinoza crowned as the good impulse because knowledge is a virtue. "Not to make a spectacle of oneself" as the wit applies to Spinoza, a lens grinder by profession, science not harnessed with some form of ethical anchor and compass can be extremely dangerous as the film *Dr. Strangelove* depicts. So why did this Goethian Faustian lovable Socrates found the scientific tradition in Nietzsche's analysis and his last words reflect a debt to medicine? Much ink has flowed in this quest which we call love of wisdom, it is not so much the end result, but the process and journey in along "the way," Hebrew: *al ha-derekh*, Greek: *hodos*, German: *auf dem Weg*, French, *penser par le methode* , Latin, *in viam cogitationis*, for thinking clears a way, to searching out human nature's secrets, and gaining hopefully not only more knowledge but a better understanding of the human beings' place in the awesome universe. There have been numerous martyrs of science and philosophy, including in the Rabbinic tradition Maimonides[74] who sought to reconcile the science of his day with Torah, a task that involved rejecting Aristotle's view of the eternality of the heavens in favor of creation *ex nihilo*, and embracing the world created in time, by a divine Being, unmoved mover, who is in time (*hu hove, huh hayah, hu yiheyeh*) yet transcends time itself, even beyond the first and last which He created in his love for goodness.

Like Iyov we are dumbfounded when God, if ever, responds out of the whirlwind to our questions,

---

[74] Levy, David B., **Censorship** of Rambam's "Sefer Madda" and "Moreh ha-Nevukhim," Association of Jewish Libraries: Annual Convention 35 (2000) 172-17.

only to be asked, "do you know the secrets of oceanography?, the secrets of geology?, the secrets of paleobiology? The secrets of animal husbandry?, the secrets of bird migrations?, the secrets of nature in general?, etc." When G-d shows up after the whirlwind, Job, whose sense of moral decency to demand justice in the world and why the innocent sometimes suffer, is mesmerized with the questions:

1 Then the LORD answered Job out of the whirlwind, and said:

ב מִי זֶה, מַחְשִׁיךְ עֵצָה בְמִלִּין-- בְּלִי-דָעַת.

2 Who is this that darkeneth counsel by words without knowledge?

ג אֱזָר-נָא כְגֶבֶר חֲלָצֶיךָ; וְאֶשְׁאָלְךָ, וְהוֹדִיעֵנִי.

3 Gird up now thy loins like a man; for I will demand of thee, and declare thou unto Me.

ד אֵיפֹה הָיִיתָ, בְּיָסְדִי-אָרֶץ; הַגֵּד, אִם-יָדַעְתָּ בִינָה.

4 Where wast thou when I laid the foundations of the earth? Declare, if thou hast the understanding.

ה מִי-שָׂם מְמַדֶּיהָ, כִּי תֵדָע; אוֹ מִי-נָטָה עָלֶיהָ קָּו.

5 Who determined the measures thereof, if thou knowest? Or who stretched the line upon it?

ו עַל-מָה, אֲדָנֶיהָ הָטְבָּעוּ; אוֹ מִי-יָרָה, אֶבֶן פִּנָּתָהּ.

6 Whereupon were the foundations thereof fastened? Or who laid the corner-stone thereof,

ז בְּרָן-יַחַד, כּוֹכְבֵי בֹקֶר; וַיָּרִיעוּ, כָּל-בְּנֵי אֱלֹהִים.

7 When the morning stars sang together, and all the sons of God shouted for joy?

ח וַיָּסֶךְ בִּדְלָתַיִם יָם; בְּגִיחוֹ, מֵרֶחֶם יֵצֵא.

8 Or who shut up the sea with doors, when it broke forth, and issued out of the womb;

ט בְּשׂוּמִי עָנָן לְבֻשׁוֹ; וַעֲרָפֶל, חֲתֻלָּתוֹ.

9 When I made the cloud the garment thereof, and thick darkness a swaddlingband for it,

י וָאֶשְׁבֹּר עָלָיו חֻקִּי; וָאָשִׂים, בְּרִיחַ וּדְלָתָיִם.

10 And prescribed for it My decree, and set bars and doors,

יא וָאֹמַר--עַד-פֹּה תָבוֹא, וְלֹא תֹסִיף; וּפֹא-יָשִׁית, בִּגְאוֹן גַּלֶּיךָ.

11 And said: 'Thus far shalt thou come, but no further; and here shall thy proud waves be stayed'?

יב הֲמִיָּמֶיךָ, צִוִּיתָ בֹּקֶר; ידעתה שחר (יִדַּעְתָּה הַשַּׁחַר) מְקֹמוֹ.

12 Hast thou commanded the morning since thy days began, and caused the dayspring to know its place;

יג לֶאֱחֹז, בְּכַנְפוֹת הָאָרֶץ; וְיִנָּעֲרוּ רְשָׁעִים מִמֶּנָּה.

13 That it might take hold of the ends of the earth, and the wicked be shaken out of it?

יד תִּתְהַפֵּךְ, כְּחֹמֶר חוֹתָם; וְיִתְיַצְּבוּ, כְּמוֹ לְבוּשׁ.

14 It is changed as clay under the seal; and they stand as a garment.

טו וְיִמָּנַע מֵרְשָׁעִים אוֹרָם; וּזְרוֹעַ רָמָה, תִּשָּׁבֵר.

15 But from the wicked their light is withholden, and the high arm is broken.

טז הֲבָאתָ, עַד-נִבְכֵי-יָם; וּבְחֵקֶר תְּהוֹם, הִתְהַלָּכְתָּ.

16 Hast thou entered into the springs of the sea? Or hast thou walked in the recesses of the deep?

יז הֲנִגְלוּ לְךָ, שַׁעֲרֵי-מָוֶת; וְשַׁעֲרֵי צַלְמָוֶת תִּרְאֶה.

17 Have the gates of death been revealed unto thee? Or hast thou seen the gates of the shadow of death?

יח הִתְבֹּנַנְתָּ, עַד-רַחֲבֵי-אָרֶץ; הַגֵּד, אִם-יָדַעְתָּ כֻלָּהּ.

18 Hast thou surveyed unto the breadths of the earth? Declare, if thou knowest it all.

יט אֵי-זֶה הַדֶּרֶךְ, יִשְׁכָּן-אוֹר; וְחֹשֶׁךְ, אֵי-זֶה מְקֹמוֹ.

19 Where is the way to the dwelling of light, and as for darkness, where is the place thereof;

כ כִּי תִקָּחֶנּוּ אֶל-גְּבוּלוֹ; וְכִי-תָבִין, נְתִיבוֹת בֵּיתוֹ.

20 That thou shouldest take it to the bound thereof, and that thou shouldest know the paths to the house thereof?

כא יָדַעְתָּ, כִּי-אָז תִּוָּלֵד; וּמִסְפַּר יָמֶיךָ רַבִּים.

21 Thou knowest it, for thou wast then born, and the number of thy days is great!

כב הֲבָאתָ, אֶל-אֹצְרוֹת שָׁלֶג; וְאוֹצְרוֹת בָּרָד תִּרְאֶה.

22 Hast thou entered the treasuries of the snow, or hast thou seen the treasuries of the hail,

כג אֲשֶׁר-חָשַׂכְתִּי לְעֶת-צָר; לְיוֹם קְרָב, וּמִלְחָמָה.

23 Which I have reserved against the time of trouble, against the day of battle and war?

כד אֵי-זֶה הַדֶּרֶךְ, יֵחָלֶק אוֹר; יָפֵץ קָדִים עֲלֵי-אָרֶץ.

24 By what way is the light parted, or the east wind scattered upon the earth?

כה מִי-פִלַּג לַשֶּׁטֶף תְּעָלָה; וְדֶרֶךְ, לַחֲזִיז קֹלוֹת.

25 Who hath cleft a channel for the waterflood, or a way for the lightning of the thunder;

כו לְהַמְטִיר, עַל-אֶרֶץ לֹא-אִישׁ-- מִדְבָּר, לֹא-אָדָם בּוֹ.

26 To cause it to rain on a land where no man is, on the wilderness, wherein there is no man;

כז לְהַשְׂבִּיעַ שֹׁאָה, וּמְשֹׁאָה; וּלְהַצְמִיחַ, מֹצָא דֶשֶׁא.

27 To satisfy the desolate and waste ground, and to cause the bud of the tender herb to spring forth?

כח הֲיֵשׁ-לַמָּטָר אָב; אוֹ מִי-הוֹלִיד, אֶגְלֵי-טָל.

28 Hath the rain a father? Or who hath begotten the drops of dew?

כט מִבֶּטֶן מִי, יָצָא הַקָּרַח; וּכְפֹר שָׁמַיִם, מִי יְלָדוֹ.

29 Out of whose womb came the ice? And the hoar-frost of heaven, who hath gendered it?

ל כָּאֶבֶן, מַיִם יִתְחַבָּאוּ; וּפְנֵי תְהוֹם, יִתְלַכָּדוּ.

30 The waters are congealed like stone, and the face of the deep is frozen.

לא הַתְקַשֵּׁר, מַעֲדַנּוֹת כִּימָה; אוֹ-מֹשְׁכוֹת כְּסִיל תְּפַתֵּחַ.

31 Canst thou bind the chains of the Pleiades, or loose the bands of Orion?

לב הֲתֹצִיא מַזָּרוֹת בְּעִתּוֹ; וְעַיִשׁ, עַל-בָּנֶיהָ תַנְחֵם.

32 Canst thou lead forth the Mazzaroth in their season? Or canst thou guide the Bear with her sons?

לג הֲיָדַעְתָּ, חֻקּוֹת שָׁמָיִם; אִם-תָּשִׂים מִשְׁטָרוֹ בָאָרֶץ.

33 Knowest thou the ordinances of the heavens? Canst thou establish the dominion thereof in the earth?

לד הֲתָרִים לָעָב קוֹלֶךָ; וְשִׁפְעַת-מַיִם תְּכַסֶּךָּ.

34 Canst thou lift up thy voice to the clouds, that abundance of waters may cover thee?

לה הַתְשַׁלַּח בְּרָקִים וְיֵלֵכוּ; וְיֹאמְרוּ לְךָ הִנֵּנוּ.

35 Canst thou send forth lightnings, that they may go, and say unto thee: 'Here we are'?

לו מִי-שָׁת, בַּטֻּחוֹת חָכְמָה; אוֹ מִי-נָתַן לַשֶּׂכְוִי בִינָה.

36 Who hath put wisdom in the inward parts? Or who hath given understanding to the mind?

לז מִי-יְסַפֵּר שְׁחָקִים בְּחָכְמָה; וְנִבְלֵי שָׁמַיִם, מִי יַשְׁכִּיב.

37 Who can number the clouds by wisdom? Or who can pour out the bottles of heaven,

לח בְּצֶקֶת עָפָר, לַמּוּצָק; וּרְגָבִים יְדֻבָּקוּ.

38 When the dust runneth into a mass, and the clods cleave fast together?

לט הֲתָצוּד לְלָבִיא טָרֶף; וְחַיַּת כְּפִירִים תְּמַלֵּא.

39 Wilt thou hunt the prey for the lioness? Or satisfy the appetite of the young lions,

מ כִּי-יָשֹׁחוּ בַמְּעוֹנוֹת; יֵשְׁבוּ בַסֻּכָּה לְמוֹ-אָרֶב.

40 When they couch in their dens, and abide in the covert to lie in wait?

מי יָכִין לָעֹרֵב, **מא** 41 Who provideth for the raven
צֵידוֹ: his prey, {N}
כִּי-יְלָדָו, אֶל-אֵל יְשַׁוֵּעוּ; when his young ones cry unto
יִתְעוּ, לִבְלִי-אֹכֶל. God, and wander for lack of
food?

The text goes on speaking and alluding to the
esoteric nature of the wonders of *ma'aseh bereshit*
(mysteries of the doings of divine Creation). Asking
Iyov if he knows the knowledge that scientists in
the fields of meteorology, atronomy, physics,
biology, chemistry, animal husbandry, medicine
and its subfields like anestheology, oceanography,
agriculture, embryology, botany, zoology, etc. and
any scientific discipline that seeks out the secrets of
G-d's creation and the laws set down in nature.
David Hume remarked "nature loves to hide,' and
with that scientists seek out her wisdom. While
science must never be smug and arrogant that it
has all answers, at least it can ask questions to
probe these mysteries and hopefully in the process
make life for human beings better. Questioning is
the piety of thought. The deeps those are of *ma'aseh
bereshit* which Rambam likens to physics and the
lofty things that are supernatural *ma'aseh
hamerkavah* which Rambam likens to metaphysics.[75]
Together they constitute the dews of resurrection, a
miracle so perhaps beyond human
comprehension,[76] that it is listed #13 in
Maimonides principles of faith, yet relatively

---

[75] For clarification see Levy, David Censorship of Rambam's
Sefer Mada and Sefer Moreh HaNevukhim. *Proceedings of the
35th Annual Association of Jewish Libraries, 35*, 172-177.

[76] See Schufreider, Gregory, The Logic of the Absurd,
Philosophy and Phenomenological Research. Vol 44, no1 (sept
1983) p. 61-83

speaking not as miraculous as the miracle of creation ex nihilo, *yesh miayin?*

It is science that seeks out secrets by offering us knowledge (*episteme*) via method which after Francis Bacon's *Organon* and Descartes *Methodes*, give clear modalities of inquiry for arriving at objective truths. In the end we may be either Nietzscheans seeking philosophy as an artistic way of life- a music practicing Socrates, or sober mathematician lost in the trance of the perfections of the circles of our thought. The last words of Archimedes (Εὕρηκα!) speak to his love of perfection in warning: Μὴ μοῦ τοὺς κύκλους τάραττε.*Mē mou tous kyklous taratte.* ("Do not disturb my circles." Mathematicians posses perhaps a truth that is more certain and pure than any other science. Mathematicians delight in solving problems, and the beauty of perfect proofs. ("Quod erat demonstrandum", "Which we had to prove" — (abbreviated as "ΟΕΔ") used by early mathematicians including Euclid and Archimedes, written at the end of a mathematical proof or philosophical argument, to signify the proof as complete. Later it became "QED" or the Halmos tombstone box symbol) There is little tolerance for sloppy and fuzzy logic. The motto over the entrance to Plato's Academy quoted in Elias's commentary on Aristotle's Categories was: Let no one without knowledge of geometry enter- Ἀγεωμέτρητος μηδεὶς εἰσίτω , *Ageōmetrētos mēdeis eisitō.* Plato according to Plutarch (Sympos., Probl VIII,2) states that G-d always geometrizes Ἀεὶ ὁ θεὸς γεωμετρεῖ, *Aei ho theos geōmetrei.* And a later mnemonic for π (pi) states: "always the great god applies geometry to everything." Ἀεὶ ὁ θεὸς ὁ μέγας γεωμετρεῖ τό σύμπαν, *Aei ho theos ho* megas geōmetrei to sympan. That many mathematicians from the ancient Pythagorians to Newton were enchanted by esoteric correlation of number and letter is encapsulated in Pythagoras' statement: Double see those who know the letters, Διπλουν ὁρῶσιν οἱ μαθόντες γράμματα., *Diploun horōsin hoi mathontes grammata*. Whether numerology (what rabbis liken to the after dinner drinks of *gematria, notricon, atbash,* and other methods of decodings of secret encryptions which God wishes to hide from the many, *ad captum vulgi,* is skeptically perceived as a game with number and letter, or rather a method of interpretation for culling esoteric wisdom will differ depending on one's inclination to Rationalism or mysticism. The Ramban holds that the whole Torah is a divine encrypted coding of Hashem's holy names.

Yet Rambam holds that mathematical truths although pristine and beautiful, are not the highest of truths. For Rambam mathematics is trumped by metaphysics [http://libguides.tourolib.org/ld.php?content_id=3994366] The highest of truth is in the realm of metaphysics or *ma'aseh merkavah*. *Ma'aseh merkavah* appears in Elijah's ascent in a "chariot of fire" where his disciple Elisha proclaims:

ט וַיְהִי כְעָבְרָם, וְאֵלִיָּהוּ אָמַר אֶל-אֱלִישָׁע שְׁאַל מָה אֶעֱשֶׂה-לָּךְ, בְּטֶרֶם, אֶלָּקַח מֵעִמָּךְ; וַיֹּאמֶר אֱלִישָׁע, וִיהִי נָא פִּי-שְׁנַיִם בְּרוּחֲךָ אֵלָי.

9 And it came to pass, when they were gone over, that Elijah said unto Elisha: 'Ask what I shall do for thee, before I am taken from thee.' And Elisha said: 'I pray thee, let a double portion of thy spirit be upon me.'

10 And he said: 'Thou hast asked a hard thing; nevertheless, if thou see me when I am taken from thee, it shall be so unto thee; but if not, it shall not be so.'

י וַיֹּאמֶר, הִקְשִׁיתָ לִשְׁאוֹל; אִם-תִּרְאֶה אֹתִי לֻקָּח מֵאִתָּךְ, יְהִי-לְךָ כֵן, וְאִם-אַיִן, לֹא יִהְיֶה.

11 And it came to pass, as they still went on, and talked, that, behold, there appeared a chariot of fire, and horses of fire, which parted them both asunder; and Elijah went up by a whirlwind into heaven.

יא וַיְהִי, הֵמָּה הֹלְכִים הָלוֹךְ וְדַבֵּר, וְהִנֵּה רֶכֶב-אֵשׁ וְסוּסֵי אֵשׁ, וַיַּפְרִדוּ בֵּין שְׁנֵיהֶם; וַיַּעַל, אֵלִיָּהוּ, בַּסְעָרָה, הַשָּׁמָיִם.

12 And Elisha saw it, and he cried: 'My father, my father, the chariots of Israel and the horsemen thereof!' And he saw him no more; and he took hold of his own clothes, and rent them in two pieces.

יב וֶאֱלִישָׁע רֹאֶה, וְהוּא מְצַעֵק אָבִי אָבִי רֶכֶב יִשְׂרָאֵל וּפָרָשָׁיו, וְלֹא רָאָהוּ, עוֹד; וַיַּחֲזֵק בִּבְגָדָיו, וַיִּקְרָעֵם, לִשְׁנַיִם קְרָעִים.

13 He took up also the mantle of Elijah that fell from him, and went back, and stood by the bank of the Jordan.

יג וַיָּרֶם אֶת-אַדֶּרֶת אֵלִיָּהוּ, אֲשֶׁר נָפְלָה מֵעָלָיו; וַיָּשָׁב וַיַּעֲמֹד, עַל-שְׂפַת הַיַּרְדֵּן.

This episode echoes in Isaiah's vision of the *merkavah* seen in the Jerusalem Temple in Haftorah Yetro (Isa. 6):

In the year of the death of King Uzziah, I saw the Lord sitting on a high and exalted throne, and His lower extremity filled the Temple.

אֽבִּשְׁנַת־מוֹת הַמֶּלֶךְ
עֻזִּיָּהוּ וָאֶרְאֶה אֶת־אֲדֹנָי
יֹשֵׁב עַל־כִּסֵּא רָם וְנִשָּׂא
וְשׁוּלָיו מְלֵאִים
אֶת־הַהֵיכָל:

Seraphim stood above for Him, six wings, six wings to each one; with two he would cover his face, and with two he would cover his feet, and with two he would fly.

שְׂרָפִים עֹמְדִים מִמַּעַל
לוֹ שֵׁשׁ כְּנָפַיִם שֵׁשׁ כְּנָפַיִם
לְאֶחָד בִּשְׁתַּיִם | יְכַסֶּה
פָנָיו וּבִשְׁתַּיִם יְכַסֶּה
רַגְלָיו וּבִשְׁתַּיִם יְעוֹפֵף:

Further in Ezekiel's vision on the Chabar river in Babylon the holy chariot of G-d is also glimpsed but this time as a reflection in the waters:

1 Now it came to pass in the thirtieth year, in the fourth month, in the fifth day of the month, as I was among the captives by the river Chebar that the heavens were opened, and I saw visions of God.

וַיְהִי בִּשְׁלֹשִׁים שָׁנָה, בָּרְבִיעִי
בַּחֲמִשָּׁה לַחֹדֶשׁ, וַאֲנִי
בְתוֹךְ־הַגּוֹלָה, עַל־נְהַר־כְּבָר;
נִפְתְּחוּ, הַשָּׁמַיִם, וָאֶרְאֶה, מַרְאוֹת
אֱלֹהִים.

2 In the fifth day of the month, which was the fifth year of king Jehoiachin's captivity,

ב בַּחֲמִשָּׁה, לַחֹדֶשׁ--הִיא הַשָּׁנָה
הַחֲמִישִׁית, לְגָלוּת הַמֶּלֶךְ יוֹיָכִין.

ג הָיֹה הָיָה דְבַר-ד' אֶל-יְחֶזְקֵאל
בֶּן-בּוּזִי הַכֹּהֵן, בְּאֶרֶץ כַּשְׂדִּים--
עַל-נְהַר-כְּבָר; וַתְּהִי עָלָיו שָׁם,
יַד-ד'.

3 the word of the LORD came expressly unto Ezekiel the priest, the son of Buzi, in the land of the Chaldeans by the river Chebar; and the hand of the LORD was there upon him.

Rambam (Guide III, 1-7) at: http://press.tau.ac.il/perplexed/chapters/chap_3_51.htm notes the vision of Ezekiel takes place in the 30th year (lamed), fourth month (daleth), and fifth day (hey) spelling laidah. Rambam also teaches that the word Chabar spelled in its permutations is: Bareikh (bless), rachav (ride), and Cherub (an angel resembling a child's face). Thus we see confirmation that Rambam holds metaphysics or *ma'aseh merkavah* is higher than mathematics and trumps normative logics. Nonetheless the 3 above source texts form the Tanakh destined and influenced subsequent reflection on the *ma'aseh merkavah* from the dead Sea scrolls of the 2nd temple,[77] Talmudic sugyot such as *arba'sheniknasu biPardes* (Hagigah 12b-14b), Hechalot traditions of the 6th and 7th century known as Hechalot Rabbati and Hechalot Zutrati, to the Ramban's Gerona circle in the time of the Rishonim, and later modern

---

[77] Baumgarten, Joseph M., 1928- "The Qumran Sabbath Song and rabbinic Merkabah traditions," *Revue de Qumran* 13,1-4 (1988) 199-213.

Hasidic texts such as the Tanya and Noam Elimelech ztsl.[78]

The physicists, also demand rigorous proof and critically demonstrative objective truths. They are often much too humble to speculate what occurred nanoseconds before the big bang. That speculation based on faith so far is for religious devotees seeking religion as a way of life (and for Jews Judaism is a religion of Law, as Leo Strauss has

[78] Kart, Don, Notes on the Studies of Merkavah mysticism and Hekhalot literature in English, Jewish Studies 52 (2017), 35-112; Van de Water, Rick, Early Rabbinic Judaism and the danger of Ezekiel , Review of Rabbinic Judaism 20,2 (2017) 168-192; דן, יוסף , מהיכלות רבתי להיכלות הזוהר : הדה-פרסונליזציה של מעשה מרכבה, מדעי היהדות 52 (תשעז) 143-162; אליאור, רחל, שירת הקודש בספרות ההיכלות והמרכבה., דחק ו (תשעו) 60-166, ; בן גדליה, מתניה יוסף, "דבש וחלב תחת לשונך" : למי, ובאיזה אופן, התירו ראשוני בעלי התוספות באשכנז את הוראת סודות התורה., מכלול א (תשעו) 127-146; לייטר, שמואל, אופיו המיסטי של מדרש שוחר טוב ושמואל בקוראי שמו (תשעו) 342-354 יט, ז.,; Vatamanu, Cătălin, Die Merkabah-Vision - eine ikonische Offenbarung der Ewigkeit Gottes., Nichts Neues unter der Sonne? (2014) 317-327; Waldman, Felicia, Maimonides' influence on Jewish European mysticism (13th-14th centuries), Ben Ever la-Arav VII (2014) 93-108; הוך, לירון, "מעשה מרכבה" בהגותם של ר' שמואל אבן תיבון ור' דוד קמחי כרקע לעיצוב גישתו הפילוסופית של אברבנאל., דעת 77 (תשעד) 123-141; צייטקין, יחיאל, קטעים מהספר מזרק כסף לר"י כספי מתוך פירושו של ר' יצחק די לאטש לפרשת בראשית., דעת 77 (תשעד) 95-121; רביב, רבקה , חזון "כבר אנש" בדניאל פרק ז במסורות ספרות חז"ל, סידרא כט (תשעד) 95-115; Herrmann, Klaus, Jewish mysticism in Byzantium : the transformation of Merkavah mysticism in 3 Enoch., Hekhalot Literature in Context (2013) 85-116; Swartz, Michael D, Mystics without minds? : Body and soul in Merkavah mysticism, Meditation in Judaism, Christianity, and Islam (2013) 33-43; Offenberg, Sara, Crossing over from Earth to Heaven : the image of the Ark and the "Merkavah" in the "North French Hebrew Miscellany"., Kabbalah 26 (2012) 135-158; Norris, Sally E., The imaginative effects of Ezekiel's "Merkavah" vision : Chagall and Ezekiel in creative discourse, Between the Text and the Canvas (2007) 80-94; Arbel, Daphna, Pure marble stones or water? : On ecstatic perception, group identity, and authority in Hekhalot and Merkavah literature., Studies in Spirituality 16 (2006) 21-38; Himmelfarb, Martha, Merkavah mysticism since Scholem : Rachel Elior's "The Three Temples"., Wege mystischer Gotteserfahrung (2006) 19-36; Davila, James R, The Dead Sea Scrolls and Merkavah mysticism, The Dead Sea Scrolls in Their Historical Context (2000) 249-264; Alexander, Philip S, Jewish elements in Gnosticism and magic c. CE 70 - c. CE 270, The Cambridge History of Judaism III (1999) 1052-1078; Arbel, Daphna, "Understanding of the heart" : spiritual transformation and divine revelations in the Hekhalot and Merkavah literature, Jewish Studies Quarterly 6,4 (1999) 320-344; Basser, Herbert W., Merkavah narrative : two paradigmatic examples, Annual of Rabbinic Judaism 2 (1999) 89-100; Elior, Rachel, The "Merkavah" tradition and the emergence of Jewish mysticism : from Temple to "Merkavah", from "Hekhal" to "Hekhalot", from priestly opposition to gazing upon the "Merkavah", Sino-Judaica (1999) 101-158; Davila, James R., 4QMess ar (4Q534) and Merkavah mysticism, Dead Sea Discoveries 5,3 (1998) 367-381; Prokopowicz, Mariusz, Hathor - "Pani Synaju" a Biblia : kilka kluczowych hipotez wokól tradycji "Merkawa" [Hathor - Lady of Sinai and the Bible; several key hypotheses around Merkavah tradition], Collectanea Theologica 66,4 (1997) 5-52; Ostow, Mortimer, The psychodynamics of "merkavah" , Ultimate Intimacy (1995) 152-180, mysticism, Herscher, Uri D, Yohanan ben Zakkai at Yavneh : merkavah and messiah, Bits of Honey (1993) 25-42; Schäfer, Peter, Merkavah mysticism and magic., Gershom Scholem's "Major Trends in Jewish Mysticism" (1993) 59-78; Wolfson, Elliot R, Yeridah la-merkavah" : typology of ecstasy and enthronement in ancient Jewish mysticism, Mystics of the Book (1993) 13-44; Wolfson, Elliot R, Merkavah traditions in philosophical garb : Judah Halevi reconsidered, Proceedings - American Academy for Jewish Research 57 (1991) 179-242; Steensgaard, Peter, Merkavah-mystikken : den ældste jødiske mystik., Mystik - den indre vej? (1990) 71-92; Swartz, Michael D, Patterns of mystical prayer in ancient Judaism : progression of themes in "Maaseh Merkavah",Society and Literature in Analysis (1990) 173-186; Wolfson, Elliot R, Letter symbolism and "Merkavah" imagery in the "Zohar", Alei Shefer (1990) 195-236.; International Conference on the History of Jewish Mysticism., International Conference on the History of Jewish Mysticism I (1987); Dan, Joseph, The religious experience of the "Merkavah", Jewish Spirituality I (1986) 289-307; Alexander, Philip S., Comparing Merkavah mysticism and gnosticism : an essay in method., Journal of Jewish Studies 35, 1 (1984) 1-18; Schäfer, Peter, New Testament and Hekhalot literature : the journey into Heaven in Paul and in Merkavah mysticism., Journal of Jewish Studies 35, 1 (1984) 19-35; Schäfer, Peter, Merkavah mysticism and rabbinic Judaism, Journal of the American Oriental Society 104,3 (1984) 537-541; Studies in Jewish Mysticism., Studies in Jewish Mysticism (1982); Gaylord, Harry E., Speculations, visions, or sermons., Journal for the Study of Judaism in the Persian, Hellenistic and Roman Period 13, 1/2 (1982) 187-194; Schniman, Lawrence H., "Merkavah" speculation at Qumran : the 4Q "Serekh Shirot 'Olat ha-Shabbat", Mystics, Philosophers, and Politicians (1982) 15-47; דן, יוסף, On] Ithamar Gruenwald, "Apocalyptic and Merkavah Mysticism" (1980), תרביץ נא, ד (תשמב) 685-691; רדלר-פלדמן, יהושע, Ithamar Gruenwald, "Apocalyptic and Merkavah Mysticism" (1980)., קרית ספר נז,א (תשמג) 35-36; Vajda, Georges, [On] Ithamar Gruenwald, "Apocalyptic and Merkavah Mysticism" (1980), Revue des Etudes Juives 140, 1/2 (1981) 217-224; Stroumsa, Guy G, [On] Ithamar Gruenwald, "Apocalyptic and Merkavah Mysticism" (1980), Numen 28,1 (1980) 107-109; Neusner, Jacob, The development of the Merkavah tradition., Journal for the Study of Judaism in the Persian, Hellenistic and Roman Period 2 (1971) 149-160; **Levy, David B, Maimonidean Controversy: Censorship of Rambam's Moreh HaNevukhim and Sefer Madah, AJL Proceedings, Washington DC;** Also see books: Scholem, Gershom, **Jewish Gnosticism, merkabah mysticism, and Talmudic tradition, New York, Jewish Theological Seminary of America, 1965; Elior, Rachel, The three temples : on the emergence of Jewish mysticism / Rachel Elior, Oxford ; Portland, Or. : Littman Library of Jewish Civilization, 2005;** Janowitz, Naomi., **The poetics of ascent [electronic resource] : theories of language in a rabbinic ascent text, Albany : State University of New York Press, c1989.; Halpern, Barruch, The Ma'aseh Merkvah Tradition in the Talmud, JSOT**

revealed). Religious persons may venture to attempt to ask the questions pertaining to WHY/ *Warum/ Pourquoi/ perché /LAMAH-MADUA?* The scientist may be much too sober and honest to take a leap of faith because it is absurd I believe it (*credo absurdum ist*) and therefore the scientists' epistemological goals are much more modest. That returns us to the question what is X. (*ti ti esti*) which allows us perhaps to attain a bit more knowledge in the ever-evolving movement of the scientific revolution(s) that function according to Kuhn along the fault seismic plate tectonics of the nature of paradigm shifts, but hopefully even more importantly a better understanding of understanding, *noesis noesis,* which is so high and so pure a state of consciousness that Maimonides incorporated this Aristotelian quest for the excellence of the life of the mind into the Jewish scientific quest.

A midrash holds Adam Rishon[79] knew all the sciences. For Maimonides *Adam Rishon* like Moshe Rabbenu were philosophers, who as prerequisites knew science. Today one might say that Oliver Sacks, as a music practicing Socrates, a neurologist with an appreciation for the whole gamut of the

---

[79] According to Maimonides, in the *Moreh Nevukhim,* Adam Kadmon was doing philosophy in Gan Eden, pure *ruhniut,* until he was seduced out of philosophizing into materiality, *gashmiut.* The course of Jewish history is to emerge from the nothingness of life reduced to pure physicality to reconstitute Adam Kadmon's state as a philosopher engaged in *noesis noesis,* the understanding of understanding, which is pure *Geist/Ruah/Esprit,* because HaShem Himself, the unmoved Mover in the Maimonidean/Aristotelian model, is pure thought who thinks Himself in a state of independent autonomous self-sufficiency of perfection. Both Rambam and Rosenzweig see *olam hazeh* as fundamentally unfinished (as *me on*) until the messianic age dawns.

humanities as well, has brought us to a neorological mental sunrise, that even goes beyond the findings of Kandel however brilliant, in *The Search for Memory*, for Sacks has shown us that science as a moral endeavor and art must work in tandem.... and that physicians must see the whole patient, and not be conscripted human beings themselves who have been truncated intellectually- morally- and spiritually by the specialization required in University curriculums in the post- modern condition that has given rise to the truncated type of "the post-modern physician." We must move into what Frost writes about as a "clearing", to see the forest for the trees, to fly on Maimonidean Eagles' wings to gain a perspective that is not myopic. To hear the hypnotic hush of the waterfall where the mysteries of the Tetragrammaton according to one tradition can be revealed once in 7 years only to students who can know on their own, and not be plagued with the mental truncation. And for this may we all experience the Nietzschian "*Coming of the Dawn*" (*Morgenröte. Gedanken über die moralischen Vorurteile*) and an Oliver Sacksian "Awakening" not just realizing with Shakespeare's Prospero that "one's library is not dukedom large enough" but that science need not be self destructive in the production of mass weapons of annihilation that politicians often are unqualified to administer, but rather redeeming and able to make us free from the false opinions in Plato's cave of Book 7 of *The Republic*. A scientist who is able to leave the cave of false opinions, as shadows on the wall, and ascend from the cave to see the light of the sun, in the ascent to the truth(s) can proclaim with Koheleth, "happy is he who has seen the light of the sun."[80] This light Rashi promises is the light stored up for the righteous in the world to come, which Maimonides in *Hilchot Teshuva* calls the *ziv shekhinah*, where the righteous bask in the shekhinah's light, and the crowns on the heads of the righteous correspond to the wisdom, understanding, and knowledge gained in this world"[81] and clearly Maimonides understood scientific knowledge as a prerequisite for higher

---

[80] Koheleth 1:6 וּמָתוֹק, הָאוֹר; וְטוֹב לַעֵינַיִם, לִרְאוֹת אֶ ת-הַשָּׁמֶשׁ; Rashi comments that the light created on the first day is the light stored up for the righteous in olam ha-bah. In Hilchot Teshuvah the Rambam holds that this light is the ziv Shekhinah in which the righteous bask in her light, and wear crowns on their heads. The crowns are directly proportional to the wisdom-understsnading-knowledge gained in olam ha-zeh. In olam ha-bah for the Rambam there is nothing physical, no eating, drinking etc. Rav Kook refers to a mystical light also with regards to the Akedat Yitchak that Avraham's act of faith brought down a sublime and esoteric light.

[81] Hilchot Teshuva 8:8
זה שקראו אותו חכמים העולם הבא לא מפני שאינו מצוי עתה וזה העולם אובד ואחר כך יבא אותו העולם. אין הדבר כן. אלא הרי הוא מצוי ועומד שנאמר אשר צפנת ליראיך פעלת וגו' ולא קראוהו עולם הבא אלא מפני שאותן החיים באין לו לאדם אחר חיי העולם הזה שאנו קיימים בו בגוף ונפש וזהו הנמצא לכל אדם בראשונה:

In the world to come, there is nothing corporeal, and no material substance; there are only souls of the righteous without bodies -- like the ministering angels... The righteous attain to a knowledge and realization of truth concerning God to which they had not attained while they were in the murky and lowly body. (Rambam, Mishneh Torah, Repentance 8)

כל נפש האמורה בענין זה אינה הנשמה הצריכה לגוף אלא צורת הנפש שהיא הדעה שהשיגה מהבורא כפי כחה והשיגה הדעות הנפרדות ושאר המעשים והיא הצורה שביארנו ענינה בפרק רביעי מהלכות יסודי התורה היא הנקראת נפש בענין זה. חיים אלו לפי שאין עמהם מות שאין המות אלא ממאורעות הגוף ואין שם גוף נקראו צרור החיים שנאמר והיתה נפש אדוני צרורה בצרור החיים. וזהו השכר שאין שכר למעלה ממנו והטובה שאין אחריה טובה והיא שהתאוו לה כל הנביאים

metaphysical knowledge (*ma'aseh merkavah*) as illustrated with the eagle's equation *of ma'aseh bereshit* with Aristotelian physics.

Maimonides' first authorship at a young age was of the mathematical work, *Sefer HaHigayon* (book on syllogisms). Other Jewish Philosophers, like Gersonides and Ramhal, authored works in logic and mathematics with the same title. The GRA is said to have translated parts of Euclids geometry into Hebrew. According to Dr. Charles Manekin,[82] Maimonides early work in logic is heavily influenced by the Greek logical tradition of Aristotle's *Posterior Analectics, Topica, and Categoria*... as well as Muslim Arabic works in Mathematics. Yet Maimonides last work, *the Guide for the Perplexed*, was viewed from the eagle's own assessment as the apex of all his life's learning. The halakhic works were sandwiched in between the earliest text on logic and the last written text in philosophy. This work in philosophy is an enchanted garden, indeed a key by which the author promises the careful reader like Yosef, who has a solid backround not only in rabbinics but sciences, to open the "gates', into which the soul may be refreshed and the mind delighted by fountains of wisdom.... That mathematical knowledge equated with Ben Zoma[83] who is referred in Pt. III, chapter 51 to being "still outside" doing higher math, is not enough to gain entrance

---

[82] Manekin wrote his dissertation on Gersonides Sefer HaHigayon at Yale which was later published in 1992. See The Logic of Gersonides : a Translation of Sefer ha-Heqqesh ha-Yashar (The Book of the Correct Syllogism) of Rabbi Levi ben Gershom with Introduction, Commentary, and Analytical Glossary Dordrecht : Springer Netherlands, 1992

[83] See http://libguides.tourolib.org/mathphilosophy

into the inner palaces of G-d, where fountains of wisdom refresh the soul and delight the mind, and angels of different ranks are said in the mushal to be lecturing on different topics. *Orhot Tzadikim* defines these topics such as the beauty of shabbos, the unity of G-d, the mysteries of creation, revelation brought before the tribunal of reason, etc. Clearly Chapter 51 part III of the Guide is within the genre of the *Hechalot* (palace) texts and later recapitulated in more recent works like *Orhot Tzadikim*. However most reception history of Maimonides locates the great eagle as a rationalist. A rationalist who says explicitly in *the Guide* not to engage in superstition, astrology, any form of *avodah zarah*[84], or to consult anthropomorphic works like *Shiur Komeh*, a Sefer Kabbalah.

May we all merit to understand a tincture of the wisdom that Maimonides is referring to in the parable (*mushal*) of chapter 51 pt. III,[85] and may we all be granted God's speed to make our journey in the quest for wisdom, understanding, and knowledge, in living a life of the mind, in living an examined life, in aspiring to supernal wisdom, and attaining perhaps a portion of those waters of salvation drawn from the wells of understanding. That human knowledge derived from scientific knowledge is feeble knowledge, compared with G-d's infinite wisdom, a reality Socrates made much ironic play in proclaiming that in reality counter to

---

[84] See Strickman, Norman, Without red strings or holy water: Maimoinides' Mishneh Torah, Brighton, MA : Academic Studies Press, 2011

[85] http://press.tau.ac.il/perplexed/chapters/chap_3_51.htm

the oracle of Delphi he knew in essence nothing (alluding to the Greek science of *meontology*).[86]

Along the way of the journey of life, whether we ever come to understand fully the significance of Schroedinger's question "*What is life?*[87]" which has undergone reappraisal by Loike and Steinberg,[88]

---

[86] http://www.h-net.org/reviews/showrev.php?id=10383

[87] Schrodinger, Erwin, What is life? : the physical aspect of the living cell ; with Mind and matter ; & Autobiographical sketches, Cambridge ; New York : Cambridge University Press, c1992; In an age of synthetic biology, extra terrestorial life forms on mars and elsewhere, and the inventions of modern Golems such as the Turing Test whereby a machine behind a door can win against the best chess player in the world... the question of "what is life is?" is in need of a reappraisal. For this reappraisal see Dr. John Stoltz-Loike for instance in: The Jewish perspective in creating human embryos using cloning technologies., Mishpachah (2016) 221-233; New biotechnological ways to begin life., B'Or Ha'Torah 24 (2016-2017) 35-46; Tampering with the genetic code of life : comparing secular and Halakhic ethical concerns, Hakirah 18 (2014) 41-58; Creating human embryos using reproductive cloning technologies, Journal of Halacha and Contemporary Society 67 (2014) 37-60; Gestational surrogacy., Hakirah 16 (2013) 113-132; Halachic challenges emerging from stem cell research., Jewish Political Studies Review 21,3-4 (2009) 133-149; Reconstituting a human brain in animals : a Jewish perspective on human sanctity., Kennedy Institute of Ethics Journal 18,4 (2008) 347-367; Ethical dilemmas in stem cell research : human-animal chimeras., radition 40,4 (2007) 28-49; Molecular genetics, evolution, and Torah principles., Torah u-Madda Journal 14 (2006-2007) 173-192; האם המשובט הוא בן-אדם?, 2004 (תשסד) שיבוט גנטי 115-122; Ma adam va-teda-ehu" : halakhic criteria for defining human beings., Tradition 37,2 (2003) 1-19; Forum: Judaism, genetic engineering, and the cloning of humans.", Torah u-Madda Journal 9 (2000); Human cloning and halakhic perspectives., Tradition 32,3 (1998) 31-46;

[88] Steinberg, Avraham, Human cloning : scientific, ethical and Jewish perspectives. Assia - Jewish Medical Ethics 3,2 (1998) 11-19

and more importantly what is eternal life and the *olam ha-bah*, the afterlife,[89] etc. is an unanswered question, for most scientists who are too honest to take the leap of faith. Wittgenstinian musings or discussion of the existence or non-existence of what is behind the logic of language:" *Wovon Mann nicht sprechen Kann daruber mußt mann schweigen* (proposition #7 TLP). Strauss urges us to return to the medieval enlightenment the likes of Maimonides, Gersonides, and the medieval rationalists, which was a superior understanding since what went wrong with the modern west as a result reflected in the dangerous consequence of the three greatest intellectual modern ideologues, Machiavelli,[90] Marx,[91] and Darwin.[92]

Machiavelli in his ends justify the means dooms politics to imitating the amorality of terrorism. Marx as a false prophet of secular messianism.[93] sheds some light on religion as an opiate of the masses, but is not religion allied with reason, a religion of reason out of the sources of Judaism, the title of Herman Cohen's *magnum opus*, more healthy truth than the drug intoxicated imaginings

---

[89] http://libguides.tourolib.org/afterlife

[90] See Strauss, Leo, Thoughts on Machiavelli, Chicago: Univ of Chicago, 1978

[91] Marx, Karl, A world without Jews, New York : Philosophical Library c1959; also see Marx on the German Jews

[92] See Jerry Bergman, The Darwin effect : its influence on Nazism, eugenics, capitalism & sexism, Green Forest, AR : New Leaf Publishing Group, Inc., [2014]; Weilkart, Richard, From Darwin to Hitler : evolutionary ethics, eugenics, and racism in Germany, New York : Palgrave Macmillan, 2006.

[93] Levin, Nora, *While the Messiah Tarried: Jewish Socialist Movements 1871-1917* NY: Schocken Books, 1977.

of false mystics? Then there is Darwin and his theory, which the Nazis applied as social darwinianism... in Selecting the Jews' Election for (S)election as the *untermentschen* and the Nazis as the uebermentschen Nordic stock. The Nazis by applying Darwinian socialism created laboratories where they engineered a controlled Hobbesian "state of nature, where life was nasty brutish and short, each against each... and the Nazis knew exactly what they were doing in applying Darwinian socialism of survival of the physically most fit. The Nazis estimation of the Jew was that of complete evil, so those Jews willing to compromise ethical and moral principles by collaborating with the forces of evil, etc. had more of a chance to "survive', thus confirming the Nazis estimation of the Jew as evil devoid of any virtue, integrity of principle, essentially scientifically engineering and creating laboratory conditions conducive to Jews stabbing other jews in the back. Jew against Jew was engineered by Nazis so that Jews who stole fellow bread rations, stole shoes at night, collaborated to hang other jews for being late to role call, or Jews who agreed to burn bodies in the camp became in the estimation of the Nazis confirmation of their assessment of the Jews as complete evil worthy of Darwinian social extinction and not fit to live. Ergo medieval iconagraphy of Jews with pitchforks and horns burning bodies in Hell was enacted in history on earth, whereby Capos were given pitchforks to turn bodies in burning pits, the confirmation of the Jews as satanic devils prevalent in medieval inconographic representations. The Nazi physicians who experimented in the most cruel and inhuman and malicious ways with Jewish "specimens" represent the full embodiment of complete radical evil and the degradation of science to the bottom. Worse than the animal species which functions merely out of instinct...and not malicious with the will to do harm.[94]

Despite this hell on earth, Resistance was to defy the Nazis and live and not become a murdered extinct race. Have we chosen to live our days wisely, and arrived at some appreciation of the vast awesomeness that should fill us with wonder at the Creation in all its gloriousness, after pondering G-d's appearance after the whirlwind in Sefer Iyov? Science tries to discover some of the laws set down by God in that creation whether they be the mathematics of the orbits of stars, the laws of gravity, the laws of thermodynamics, the laws of entropy, the Einsteinian laws of Relativity, and today the preoccupation with string theory and unified field theories. That we see God's footsteps and traces in His universe hopefully as Maimonides urges will fill us with wonder, fear, and love for the Creator of all that exists. Science is no religion. Science is a culture. And it remains a question whether culture can ultimately be a teleologically ultimately redemptive way of life, for it is only when we aspire to ethical cultures that culture can have a chance as autonomous knowledge that is redemptive. When we understand how science can reveal the wonder of God's work, filling us with awe and love of the Creator, his Creation, and the object of his thought-as knower, and thing known. Einstein was perhaps

---

[94] Pastermak, Alfred, Inhuman research : medical experiments in German concentration camps, Budapest : Akadémiai Kiadó, c2006 ; Baumslag, Naomi, Murderous medicine : Nazi doctors, human experimentation, and typhus, Westport, Conn. : Praeger Publishers, c2005 ; Aly, Goetz, Cleansing the fatherland : Nazi medicine and racial hygiene, Baltimore: JHU Press, 1994

right- God does not play dice, one does not have time to waste gambling their life away, and may we all be blessed to strive to cultivate an art of leisure, in a culture of redemption, that leads to Oliver Sacksian AWAKENINGS, in the expansion of our consciousness, in the expansion of our understanding of understanding. Life is worth living in any form (perhaps Socrates was wrong that the unexamined life is not worth living[?][95"]) as physicians strive to preserve the quality and longevity of life, but it is up to each person as part of an ethical community to strive to live a life of intellectual-moral-spiritual virtue, an examined life full of love for the true, the good, and the beautiful, that takes one's soul spark into something greater than their self, into something not finite, into something that is truly perpetually eternal, substantive and essential for a knowing that the journey is a gift that we must choose to find our bearings by ethical behaviors that serve the needs of others, and that by serving others, we enter into the true dignity and nobility for which man was created as a thinking-ethical-spiritual being capable of a link with G-d thru the Maimonidean active intellect informed by moral praxis. As Koheleth notes: happy is the one who has seen the light of the sun, the light of the first day which from Rashi to Rambam is understood as the *ohr genus, ohr nistarah, ohr penimit.*

Maimonides, & A. Schweitzer make medicine an ethical calling in total commitment to serving the needs of others *lifnei misharat ha-din, middoth*

---

95   The unexamined life is not worth living (Plato, Apology of Socrates 38a) -> Ο δ' ανεξέταστος βίος ου βιωτός ανθρώπω, Ὁ δ' ἀνεξέταστος βίος οὐ βιωτὸς ἀνθρώπῳ

hassiduth.[96] Rambam's devotion to his patients is attested when Rabbi Yehudah Ibn Tibbon asked when they could meet to discuss translation of the Guide from Arabic into Hebrew. The Rambam writes:

"Do not expect to be able to confer with me on any scientific subject for even one hour, either by day or by night, for the following is my daily occupation/routine: I dwell in Fostat and the Sultan resides in Cairo; these two places are two Sabbath days' journey distant form each other. My duties to the sultan are very heavy. I am obliged to visit him every day, early in the morning; and when he or any of his children, or any of the inmates of his harem are indisposed, I dare not quit Kahira, but must stay during the greater part of the day in the palace. It also frequently happens that one or two royal officers fall sick, and I must attend to their healing. Hence, as a rule, I repair to Kahira very early in the day, and even if nothing unusual happens, I do not return to Fostat until the afternoon. Then I am almost dying with hunger. I find the antechambers filled with people, both Jews

---

[96] Acting beyond the letter of the law is a technical halakhic category in Jewish law. Louis Jacobs has argued that this radical ethic of selfless altruistic love can be found *deoreita* from the cases of: (1) Zebulon and Naphtali (Judges 5:18), (2) Abraham's risking of his life to save Lot (Gen.16:14-16), (3) Lot risking his life to shelter two angels (Gen.12:10-20), (4) Moshe risking his life by smiting the Egyptian (Ex.2:11-15), (5) Moshe offering his life in prayer as intercession (Ex.32:32), (6) Moshe risking his life by delivering the daughters of Jethro (Ex. 2:17-19), (7) Samson killing himself in order to slay Philistines (Judges 16:28-30), (8) David placing his life in jeopardy when accepting the challenge of Goliath (I.Sam.17), or *derabbanan* in Pesahim 25b, Terumot 8:12, and Pesahim 50a. See L. Jacobs, "Greater Love Hath No Man...The Jewish Point of View of Self-Sacrifice", *Judaism* 6.1 (1957

and Gentiles, nobles and common people, judges and bailiffs, friends and foes- a mixed multitude who await the time of my return. I dismount from my animal, wash my hands, go forth to my patients, and entreat them to bear with me while I partake of some slight refreshment, the only meal I take in the 24 hours. Then I go forth to attend to my patients, and write prescriptions and directions for their various ailments. Patients go in and out until nightfall, and sometimes even I solemnly assure you until two hours or more in the night. I converse with and prescribe for them while lying down from sheer fatigue; and when night falls, I am so exhausted that I can scarcely speak. In consequence of this, no Israelite can have any private interview with me, except on Sabbath. On that day the whole congregation or at least the majority of the members come to me after the morning service, when I instruct them as to their proceedings during the whole week; we study together a little until noon, when they depart. Some of them return and read with me after the _minchah_ until _ma'ariv_. In this manner I spend that day. I have here related to you only a part of what you would see if you were to visit me."

Marx, "Texts by and about Maimonides," 378, Jewish Quarterly Review, 25, 1925, p. 371-428. (MS Adler recension)

The ideal physician is devoted to serving the needs of patients to enhance longevity and quality of life, to do no harm…. (Hippocrates) And alleviate pain & distress. Ergo the physicians leisure time is often non-existent- in the calling to serve the needs of others.

For Dr. Robert I Levy serving patients is a calling and not merely a professional job, and that meant being on call 24/6 and frequently being called out at 3 am. in the morning to save lives, and making house calls acting *lifnei mishrat ha-din, middoth hasiduth*. G-d tells Abraham, *"He'yeh bracha"* - "You shall be a blessing." It doesn't say "You shall be *blessed*, but you shall be a blessing, teaching us that the greatest gift to which we can aspire is to be *a blessing to others*, to be able to make a difference in their lives, and if we can do that, even during massive snow storms Dr. Robert Levy was often seen trudging thru snow and ice when roads were not drivable, to arrive at Sinai hospital to make sure his patients were receiving proper care. Further Dr. Levy made countless thousands of *pro bonum* house calls to shut ins in remote areas sometimes 5 hours drive from Baltimore city, airing out apartments-making personal trips to get the patients medicines at the local drug stores sometimes another mile away from their remote isolated residence, and making sure they had care lined up with nurses for the future, paying out of pocket personally when the patients could not afford the in house nurse services. In the age when patients were not kicked out of the hospitals in 5 days. A certain case involved a man who came to Sinai hospital. at a time when the weather was nice and warm...but a month later released to a snowy icy landscape, not only did Dr. Levy (bis hundert und zwanzig, personally escort the patient to the cab, paying for his transit home, but actually went back to the house to retrieve a winter coat, gloves, and ski cap for the patient who had only brought summer shorts and t-shirt to the hospital before his stay etc. There are countless examples of Dr. Levy's devotion, and caring commitment to serve his patients. Dr. Levy continues to do *Bikur holim* visits every week at local Baltimore hospitals, totally *pro bonum...* in his retirement. Dr. Levy understands that human life has no price tag, and is infinite worth as the rabbis note everyone is a world and thus we wear tzizit.., etc. not just to remind us not to go after the assumptions of the eyes, but because the body is likened to the "4 corners of the world" and everyone is a microcosm for the macrocosm....

וכל המקיים נפש אחת מישראל מעלה עליו הכתוב כאילו קיים עולם מלא ומפני שלום הבריות

Even if Dr. Rosner[97] ascribes Maimonides prayer to the *apres la lettre* to the 17th Century there is still much we can learn from it, and see it as a noble embodiment for all physicians in the legacy of Maimonides, with a sense of the noble devotion endowed in medicine to cure the sick with recognition of G-d as the ultimate healer. There we read:

> *Almighty God, Thou has created the human body with infinite wisdom. Ten thousand times ten thousand organs hast Thou combined in it that act unceasingly and harmoniously to preserve the whole in all its beauty the body which is the envelope of the immortal soul. They are ever acting in perfect order, agreement and accord. Yet, when the frailty of matter or the unbridling of passions deranges this order or interrupts this accord, then forces clash and the body crumbles into the primal dust from which it came. Thou sendest to man diseases as*

---

[97] Rosner, Fred, The physician's prayer attributed to Moses Maimonides, Bulletin of the History of Medicine 41 (1967) 440-454

beneficent messengers to foretell approaching danger and to urge him to avert it.

Thou has blest Thine earth, Thy rivers and Thy mountains with healing substances; they enable Thy creatures to alleviate their sufferings and to heal their illnesses. Thou hast endowed man with the wisdom to relieve the suffering of his brother, to recognize his disorders, to extract the healing substances, to discover their powers and to prepare and to apply them to suit every ill. In Thine Eternal Providence Thou hast chosen me to watch over the life and health of Thy creatures. I am now about to apply myself to the duties of my profession. Support me, Almighty God, in these great labors that they may benefit mankind, for without Thy help not even the least thing will succeed.

Inspire me with love for my art and for Thy creatures. Do not allow thirst for profit, ambition for renown and admiration, to interfere with my profession, for these are the enemies of truth and of love for mankind and they can lead astray in the great task of attending to the welfare of Thy creatures. Preserve the strength of my body and of my soul that they ever be ready to cheerfully help and support rich and poor, good and bad, enemy as well as friend. In the sufferer let me see only the human being. Illumine my mind that it recognize what presents itself and that it may comprehend what is absent or hidden. Let it not fail to see what is visible, but do not permit it to arrogate to itself the power to see what cannot be seen, for delicate and indefinite are the bounds of the great art of caring for the lives and health of Thy creatures.

Let me never be absent-minded. May no strange thoughts divert my attention at the bedside of the sick, or disturb my mind in its silent labors, for great and sacred are the thoughtful deliberations required to preserve the lives and health of Thy creatures.

Grant that my patients have confidence in me and my art and follow my directions and my counsel. Remove from their midst all charlatans and the whole host of officious relatives and know-all nurses, cruel people who arrogantly frustrate the wisest purposes of our art and often lead Thy creatures to their death.

Should those who are wiser than I wish to improve and instruct me, let my soul gratefully follow their guidance; for vast is the extent of our art. Should conceited fools, however, censure me, then let love for my profession steel me against them, so that I remain steadfast without regard for age, for reputation, or for honor, because surrender would bring to Thy creatures sickness and death.

Imbue my soul with gentleness and calmness when older colleagues, proud of their age, wish to displace me or to scorn me or disdainfully to teach me. May even this be of advantage to me, for they know many things of which I am ignorant, but let not their arrogance give me pain. For they are old and old age is not master of the passions. I also hope to attain old age upon this earth, before Thee, Almighty God!

Let me be contented in everything except in the great science of my profession. Never allow the *thought to arise in me that I have attained to sufficient knowledge, but vouchsafe to me the strength, the leisure and the ambition ever to extend my knowledge. For art is great, but the mind of man is ever expanding.*

Almighty God! Thou hast chosen me in Thy mercy to watch over the life and death of Thy creatures. I now apply myself to my profession. Support me in this great task so that it may benefit mankind, for without Thy help not even the least thing will succeed.[98]

Even if such a physician's prayer is an anachronism in the history of medicine, perhaps the Rambam would be touched by its content and recognize in it the humility from which a physician is a servant of G-d placed on the earth to heal, care for, and promote longevity and quality of life for the benefit of all mankind, doing no harm, and eliminating pain.

וַיִּקַּח ד' אֱלֹהִים, אֶת-הָאָדָם; וַיַּנִּחֵהוּ בְגַן-עֵדֶן, לְעָבְדָהּ וּלְשָׁמְרָהּ.	15 And the LORD God took the man, and put him into the garden of Eden to care for it and to safekeep it.

Today the medical field has a role to play in returning the fallen state of human beings to their Edenic state in the garden, but for instance eliminating the pains of childbirth through epidurals given to women in labor. Further Bio-technology have the potential to reverse the evil of

[98] translated by Harry Friedenwald, Bulletin of the Johns Hopkins Hospital 28: 260-261, (1917)

disease and the suffering it causes through various methods such as stem cell research, cloning, and genetic engineering which may one day in the future prove to eliminate genetic diseases with the ease by which one photocopies.

A new day is perhaps dawning spoke of in the midrash when the sun's light will become equal to that of the moon's light representing the shekhinah. Lurianic Kabbalah claims that the 2 orot, shemesh veyareach, and the 1st 2 humans, Adam and Chava, male and female aspects of the Godhead were equal in the embryonic stage of *ma'aseh bereshit*. However as a result of the exit from Eden the *lavanah* became smaller and the *Shechinah* went into *Galut*. It is only in *geulah* that the 2 will be restored to their rightful places. A similar destiny is promised women and technology may play a role in that. For example biomedical technology allows women to give birth at older ages and with less labor pain. Organ transplantations, fertility treatments allowing spouses to have children at older ages, and stomping out disease and suffering makes science at the forefront of potentially redeeming the world towards a restoration of its more Edenic origin. The imperative to heal, cure, care for, and promote quality of life recognizes the dignity and sanctification of G-d's creatures and constitutes a Kiddush Hashem by helping play as a partner in enhancing and increasing the greatest gift of all quality of life. Physicians like the Rambam, however rare they be, prefer to earn a *parnasah* engaged in this sacred endeavor of the mission and calling of medicine, divorced from any selfagrandisement, egotism, solipsism, greed, avarice, or negative vices, for the benefit and good the sacred art of healing can bring to the world and human beings. The eight blessing of the Amidah states:

> Heal us, O L-rd, and we will be healed; help us and we will be saved; for You are our praise. Grant complete cure and healing to all our wounds; for You, Almighty King, are a faithful and merciful healer. Blessed are You L-rd, who heals the sick of His people Israel.

Thus it is the physician who as a *shaliach* of *refuah* works on behalf of G-d to sanctify life by helping give the greatest gift which is life itself endowing human beings with being *Bitzelem Elokim*, as Rambam notes possessing potential for attaining intellectual-moral-spiritual virtue in *olam ha-zeh* which rebounds directly proportional to one's threefold accomplishments in *olam ha-bah* where the righteous bask in the *ziv shekhinah*.

Table of Contents

Chapter One

History of Sinai Hospital in Baltimore, Maryland

History of Sinai Hospital 1863-2009: Its Place in the
History of Jewish Hospitals in America

Introduction

Webster's dictionary indicates that the word
hospital is derived from the Latin, *hospitalis–of a
guest, hospes–guest)*. Indeed a hospital in the late
eighteenth century and early nineteenth centuries
in America were very much an almshouse, a
residence for the poor.[1] At the turn of the
nineteenth century only the Philadelphia
Pennsylvania Hospital, founded in 1752 and the

New York Hospital founded in 1771 could be considered a "hospital" as an institution dedicated exclusively to inpatient care of the sick."[1] The Boston Massachusetts General Hospital opened in 1821. Well established hospital in Europe in Edinburgh, Scotland and Paris in the eighteenth century and early in the nineteenth century Guys Hospital in London were already in operation in larger populations than the five million who lived in all of America in 1800 and only 320,000 of these lived in communities larger than twenty-five hundred.[2] "In 1800 the hospital was still an insignificant aspect of American medical care. No gentleman of property or standing would have found himself in a hospital unless stricken with insanity or felled by epidemic or accident in a strange city."[3]

In the period 1800-1850 the hospitals in Europe, England and especially France, replacing Edinburgh, made considerable progress in advancement of medical knowledge and care attracting may privileged Americans who flocked especially to Paris. On returning these "antebellum hospitals remained the professional domain of a (this) small medical elite, irrelevant to the care of the vast majority of Americans and to the careers o of those practitioners who treated them."[4] Medicine

---

[1] Rosenberg, Charles E., The Care of Strangers, The Rise of America's Hospital System, 1987, p. 4.

[2] U.S. Bureau of the Census, Historical Statistics of the United States, Colonial Times to 1970.

[3] Rosenberg, Charles E. , The Care of Strangers, The Rise of American's Hospital System, 1987. p. 4.

[4] Ibid, p. 70.

as practiced by the majority of American physicians remained rudimentary, limited to observation of the pulse, character of the tongue, and noting the number of diarrheal stools. Medication was also limited to the eighteenth century practice of bleeding, cupping, and purging. Hospitals in most cities were almshouses for care of chronically ill, indigent, and foreign born.[5]

It was on May 10th 1863, during the Civil War and the year of the battle of Gettysburg, that Mr. Rayner of the Hebrew Benevolent Society of Baltimore (a forerunner of the Associated Jewish Charities) called a meeting of the community to discuss the need of founding a hospital directed toward the needs of the then expanding German orthodox Jewish Community.[6]

Overview of Jewish Hospitals in Europe

Alan M. Kraut, Professor of History at The American University in Washington, D.C., has summarized the development of Jewish Hospital in Europe and America:

"Jewish hospitals have a venerable history arising form the twin traditions of community self help and resistance

---

[5] The Baltimore Almshouse occupied the area where Johns Hopkins now is located, across the street from the eventual location of the Hebrew Hospital and Asylum.

[6] History of Sinai Hospital, Eugene J. Leopold, M.D. Chairman of the Medical Board, from School of Nursing Announcement, Winnie A.Coxe, R.N. Director of Nurses and Principal of the School of Nursing, 1943. Also see Sinai Hospital of Baltimore, Inc. Centennial Anniversary Paper Presented by Mrs. M. Sigmund Shapiro at Annual Meeting of Jewish Historical Society, May 8,1966

to anti-Semitism. Evidence suggests that as early as the eleventh century[7], synagogues in cities such as Cologne had one room, a **hekdesh,** reserved for the care of sick itinerants. By the eighteenth century, little had changed in most communities other that to relocate the **Hekdesh,** outside the town, often near a cemetery. Rarely were there more than two rooms with a few beds in each room. If most who came could not be cured, at least they could die with dignity in the care of coreligionists. More elaborate facilities, **Krankenhausen,** or "houses for the sick," were erected in larger Western European cities. A 250 bed hospital opened in Breslau in 1726; two decades later, London's Sephardic community opened another: and by the end of the century, Berlin and Vienna opened still others. The first Jewish hospital in Paris opened its doors in 1836, followed by Amsterdam in 1840 and Hamburg in 1841. In Jerusalem, the Mayer de Rothschild Hospital was established in the Old City in 1854. Jewish hospitals appeared in Eastern Europe, as well. By the first third of the twentieth century, forty-eight hospitals in Poland identified themselves as Jewish, including a one-thousand-bed facility in Warsaw." [8]

Overview of Jewish Hospitals in America

Professor Alan Kraut continues with an overview of the development of Jewish Hospitals in America: "In the United states, early Jewish communities cared for their own from death to life. The first community effort of Jewish settlers in a city was to form a burial society to purchase land for a Jewish cemetery. There,

---

[7]

[8] Kraut Alan M. and Deborah A. Kraut, Covenant of Care Newark Beth Israel and The Jewish Hospital in America. Rutgers University Press, 2006, p.2.

Jews could be buried with other of their faith. Hebrew Benevolent Societies composed of merchants and businessmen soon undertook additional responsibilities, including the founding of orphanages and the provision of institutions for invalids.[9] (Such an 'Asylum for Hebrew Children' was established in West Baltimore, to be described later)

"The first U.S. Jewish hospitals emerged in response to urban epidemics of cholera or yellow fever in the mid-nineteenth century. In the 1849 cholera epidemic in Cincinnati, a commercial city populated by German Jewish merchants and craftspeople, spurred the founding of Jewish Hospital a year later. Jewish Hospital was intended by its founders to serve the approximately four thousand Jew who lived in the city, as well as impoverished and homeless peddlers who moved from place to place though the Midwest and clung to their Jewish identities.

New York City, ravaged by waves of cholera, in 1852 chartered the Jews' Hospital (renamed Mount Sinai during the Civil War). After three years of fund-raising, much of it personally guided by businessman Samson Simson, the hospital open its doors in 1855 "for the purpose of affording surgical and medical aid, comfort and protection in sickness to deserving and needy Israelites for the purposes appertaining to hospital and dispensaries, a benevolent, charitable and scientific hospital."

In 1868, another businessman, Judah Touro, in yellow fever-infected New Orleans, spearheaded the founding of a Jewish hospital that took his name.

---

[9] Ibid., p.3

After an epidemic of typhoid fever, the German Jew who had come to San Francisco as peddlers and shopkeepers during the Gold Rush founded the Mount Zion Hospital Association.

In Chicago, the rebuilding of the city after the great fire of 1871 included the construction of Michael Reese Hospital named for the Bavarian-born businessman whose family inherited the fortune he had amassed in San Francisco. Reese's family donated his legacy to build a Jewish hospital in Chicago and his relatives sustained the legacy by continuing to support its expansion."[10]

Professor Kraut in his Introduction to *Covenant of Care* goes on to explain how the Manhattan's Mount Sinai was joined with a variety of other hospitals including Montefiore and other Jewish hospital formed in Brooklyn. He points out that hospitals named Sinai were formed in Los Angeles, Cleveland and Philadelphia. The name "Jewish Hospital" was used in Louisville and St. Louis.[11]

Early History of Medical Care and Hospitals in Maryland

The Baltimore Almshouse was established in 1773 and moved to a converted private dwelling in Calverton in 1822. Its occupants were primarily paupers caring for the sick and chronically ill.[12] The Bay View Asylum, overlooking the

---

[10] Ibid. p.3-4.

[11] Ibid, p

[12] See Douglas, Carroll (a physician graduated from the University of Maryland Medical School who worked at the Baltimore Almshouse in 1834) Medical Students 1818 and 1838, Maryland State Medical Journal (February 1974): 40

Chesapeake, built in 1866 received the Almshouse inmates, assuming the responsibility of caring for the city's poor. A quarantine hospital was established in 1797 to safeguard the city from infectious diseases entering the port at Hawkins Point. The Maryland Hospital was founded in 1797 as a lunatic and general hospital.[13] This hospital cared for private patients who paid three to five dollars a week and public patients who were supported by the state. In 1872 Spring Grove in Catonsville opened to care for the growing number of mental patients. As a teaching arm of the University of Maryland Medical School the Baltimore Infirmary was established in 1823 at the corner of Lombard and Greene Streets. After the Civil War the Infirmary expanded greatly. As the number of immigrants entering the city increased additional hospitals having religious backing were established, Union Protestant Infirmary (Union Memorial) in 1854, St. Joseph's in 1864, and St Agnes in 1878. The Hebrew Hospital in Baltimore was an additional sectarian hospital to be established in 1863.

Background for the Establishment of a Jewish Hospital in Baltimore

The Early German Jews of Baltimore

A lecture by Moses Aberbach[14] delivered to the Society for the History of the Germans of

---

[13] Troy, John D., Report of the President and Board of Visitors of the Maryland Hospital, 1851, pp.18-23.

[14] Aberbach, Moses, The Early Gernan Jews of Baltimore, Lecture delivered to the Society for the History of the Germans of Maryland, February 18, 1970.

Maryland, in February 28, 1970 is the source of the following information on the German Jews who represented the   initial Jewish community of Baltimore. These immigrant Jews of Baltimore were overwhelmingly of Bavarian origin before the Civil War. While there was a handful of Sephardic and eastern European Jews, the Jewish community of Baltimore in these early days almost exclusively consisted of orthodox German Jews from Bavaria. The Jews of Bavaria were oppressed and not granted citizenship and treated with disdain. With the conquest of the area by Napoleon in 1806 the Jews were granted some rights, attending government schools, serving in the army , but at the expense of elimination of Rabbinic courts dealing with disputes, marriage and divorce. The Jews continued to plead for more rights and full emancipation without success. Even following the revolution of 1848 continued appeals for emancipation were ignored and immigration to the United States which had begun even earlier was accelerated. As noted by Moses Aberbach, "Every wave of Jewish immigration to Baltimore up to the period of the Civil War was directly due to the intolerable situation of Bavarian Jewry." Baltimore was chosen as the port of entry to the United States because the shipping companies , handling wheat and tobacco, induced them to come. The ships carrying these goods from America to Europe, not having other cargo to send back to America, returned baring people, mostly poor people. Aberbach indicates that the male immigrants would often return to Bavaria, not to resettle back home but to obtain a young bride. Such was the actions of one of Baltimore's leading early Rabbis, Benjamin Szold, whose daughter was an important factor on Hadassah and Israel in years to come.

The two wealthy families of Etting and Cohen, while regarding themselves as aristocratic Sephardim, where important in encouraging Thomas Kennedy, originally from Scotland and settling in Hagerstown, to obtain support for the so called Jew Bill. Kennedy while coming to America as a poor immigrant had become a member of the Maryland legislature. This Jew Bill in 1826 after a number of years and failed attempts in the Legislature and with the help of Thomas Kennedy allowed the Jewish population of Maryland to obtain full rights and privileges of citizenship, holding office, practicing a profession and voting that they never had in Bavaria and allowed. This bill also allowed a Jewish Hospital in Baltimore to be established thirty six years later in 1863. A large 3 by 5 foot marble plaque recognizing Thomas Kennedy efforts in passage of this Jew Bill was to be found between the elevators, where it could be easily seen by all visitors to the "old Sinai" hospital on Monument Street and currently rests in the "memorabilia section" of the current hospital but in a less conspicuous space than previously.

Early History of Sinai Hospital of Baltimore

While the first hospitals sponsored by Jewish people in Cincinnati and New York were initiated by the response to urban epidemics of cholera in 1849 and 1852 respectively, the need for such a hospital in Baltimore to serve the Jewish Community was more related to 1. the lack of the Kosher diet in other facilities not conforming to the Jewish Dietary laws, 2. Jews dying unattended by co-religionist as well as the concern of Dr. Aaron

Friedenwald 3. "that young Jewish doctors should be as well trained as their non-Jewish colleagues", training and experience being limited in the non Jewish community.[15] "The death of a young Jew in a general hospital in 1863, unattended by his co-religionist, brought the question to the fore."

To quote from the paper of Dr. Eugene J. Leopold of 1943, " Finally on May 10th 1863, Mr. Rayner of the Hebrew Benevolent Society called a meeting of the community. The problem of founding a hospital was presented. Immediately 46 men pledged $1948.00 toward a Hospital Building Fund. It had been estimated that a suitable ten room building would cost $10,000.00 and annual cost of maintenance would be $1,280.00. Soon thereafter, Mr. Samuel B. Ellinger offered a plot of ground for the proposed Hospital and Mr. Sutton a house and lot on Locus Street. But neither was accepted, as the location was not suitable. At the meeting in May 1863, a Building Committee had been appointed which, after some changes consisted of Henry Straus, Chairman, Julius Stiefel, Dr. Joshua I. Cohen, Moses Oettinger, Samuel Ellinger, Jonas Friedenwald, Jacob Hecht, M. Hirschberg, A Rosenfield and Wiesenfeld. *This committee was offered a plot of ground facing 200 feet on Monument Street, and running back 150 feet on Ann Street (now*

---

[15] History of Sinai Hospital, Eugene J. Leopold, 1943, p. 1.

Rutland Ave)[16]. It was opposite the grounds of the Mayland Asylum, where now stands the Johns Hopkins Hospital. It lay on the outskirts of the City, and would cost $2100.00. This was considered a suitable site for the proposed Hospital.[17] (see map of relationship of Johns Hopkins and "Asylum for Israelites" an alternative name for the Hebrew Hospital and Asylum Association, the designated name of the Hospital until 1926 when the name was changed to Sinai Hospital of Baltimore).

To quote from the paper of Mrs. M. Sigmund Shapiro from 1966,[18] " In 1863, then a resolution to build a hospital was adopted by the Hebrew Benevolent Society. The lot on which the old Sinai Hospital stood was, at that time occupied by the city poorhouse. This property was purchased, for the sum of $2100, (as noted above) by Samuel Ellinger, Jacob Hecht, Henry and Levi Straus, as was donated to the Hebrew Benevolent Society. *The*

---

[16] Ann Street was named along with Bond Street were named and marked out by Mr. Fell of Fells Point. He married Ann Bond and called these streets after his wife, Ann and Bond Streets. Ann street ran north from Fells Point across the area where Hopkins is now situated, being the eastern boarder of the Maryland Asylum, from where came Siania's first patient, Jacob Schwetzer (see below) and proceed north to Boundary Ave, the northern boundry of the City. Boundary Ave is currently North Ave. Ann Street is a lovely street currently south of Hopkins which intercepted its original progress and Ann Street north of Monument St. was named Hopkins Way and then Rutland Ave which is its current designation but only for a block.

[17] History of Sinai Hospital , Eugene J. Leopold , p. 1

[18] Sinai Hospital of Baltimore, Inc. Centennial Anniversary Paper, Presented by Mrs. Sigmund Shapiro at Annual Meeting of the Jewish Historical Society. P. 1-2

cornerstone of the building was laid on June[19] 25, 1866. All in all, it took five years from the date of the resolution to erect the hospital which began as a ten room home." (See drawing of original 10 room hospital) Financing as today was the major factor in the delay of its construction.

Mrs. Shapiro continues in her report of May 8, 1966, "The total cost of the building was about $60,000 of which $17,500 was raised by a 'Fair' which was held in the Concordia Opera House. The "Fair was sponsored by the Ladies Auxiliary, of which Mrs. Betsey Weisenfeld was president." Eugene Leopold's *History of Sinai Hospital* from 1943 indicates the funds for this 10 room building were obtained from additional sources as well, " Various and many picnics, Fairs, and amateur Theatrical performances resulted in adding to the funds by from $50.00 to $200.00 each, making the fund $10,5636. 00 including $3000.00 lent by the Hebrew Benevolent Society, which was anxious to reinvest its funds."[20]

Mr. Leopold[21] in his report of 1943 pointed out that in 1826, the same year as the "Bill of Rights" law introduced by Thomas Kennedy finally became a law and the Jews of Baltimore acquired the "right to vote and hold office", The Baltimore Hebrew Congregation , became the first organized Temple in Baltimore. As an out growth of this organization's interest in charitable as well as

---

[19] Ibid., p.1

[20] Ibid. p. 2.

[21] History of Sinai Hospital, Eugene J. Leopold, M.D. Chairman of the Medical Board, prepared for the School of Nursing Announcement in 1943. p. 1.

religious activities, there was formed in 1846 the Hebrew Assistance Society, a forerunner of the Associated Jewish Charities. Ten years later in 1856 merging with several smaller organizations there was formed the Hebrew Benevolent Society, which became a prominent factor in charitable contribution to the founding of Hebrew Hospital and Asylum.

Finally on May 17, 1868 plans were made for the dedication of the new hospital. According to Mr. Leopold, "the dedication ceremonies were postponed until May 24, 1968 because of rain. The Dedication ceremonies began with music by Professor Winters band, then came prayers for the success of the undertaking by Rev. A. Leucht. After which M. Joseph Friedenwald mad an eloquent address, which was followed by an address in German by Rev. H. Hochheimer and closing prayer by Dr. B. Zzold. There was music between speeches, by a choir of 24 males and 12 female voices singing several hymns. During the ceremonies a collection had been in progress which was presented as a token of thanks at the conclusion of the ceremonies which totaled #1848.25. It must have been a very happy and pleasing affair, although very long." Paul Umansky[22] has written *Story of Sinai Hospital, 1866-1959* in July, 1997, for *Reflections*, a publication of the Jewish Museum of Maryland and notes that, "The cornerstone for this Baltimore Asylum for Israelites was laid in 1866 and a tattered, blue-covered little volume (one or two others are extant, in different color covers) shows that five speeches

---

[22] Umansky , Paul, Story of Sinai Hospital, 1866, -1959, written in July 1997 for Reflections, a publication of the Jewish Museum of Maryland, p. 1and 2.

ere delivered at this ceremony, three in English and two in German, which should tell you where many of Baltimore's Jewish immigrant were coming from." Mr. Umansky goes on to relate that, "An inconspicuous article in the The Sun of the day tells us that '....a large number of persons attended, the greater portion being Israelites."

And what about the first patient to the Hebrew Hospital and Asylum, also referred to a Sheltering Home. Mr. Leopold again provides us with the details:[23]

"Meanwhile, where had been received an application for admission. A Mr. Jacob Schwetzer, an inmate across the street, in the Maryland Asylum suffering with 'consumption', wrote a postal card asking admittance to the Hebrew Hospital where 'he might get a diet better suited to his disease'. A committee of two 'Managers' was sent to see Mr. Schwetzer, they reported him ill, without money or friends. Then Dr. A.B. Arnold was sent to examine him. He reported Mr. Schwetzer 'a suitable case for admission as seen as suitable quarters could be arranged for him. Thus Jacob. Schwetzer became the first patient of the Hebrew Hospital. "

This was on 5/3/1868 as recorded in the Record Book of the Hebrew Hospital and Asylum Association. (see below for details)

---

[23] Leopold, Eugene J. M.D. History of Sinai Hospital , Chairman of the Medical Board,1943, p. 3

Early History of the Hebrew Hospital and Asylum
(otherwise known as Asylum for Israelites)

Hospitals in America, few in number just following the Civil War functioned very differently than those today or even by the turn of the twentieth century. Charles E. Rosenberg points out that, " In our country, as the mid-nineteenth-century New Yorker magazine put it, 'the people who repair to hospitals are mostly very poor, and seldom go into them until driven to do so from a severe stress of circumstances' " [24] Only a few hospitals at that time such as the Philadelphia Pennsylvania Hospital, New York Hospital and the Massachusetts General Hospital in Boston could be considered dedicated to inpatient care of the sick. The Hebrew Hospital and Asylum was in these early years more an Asylum or Almshouse than a hospital in the modern sense. To quote Rosenberg again,

"The hospital was not yet dominated and justified, as it has come to be, by an intimidating arsenal of tolls and techniques. Aside from a handful of tools and techniques. Aside from a handful of surgical procedures, there was little in the way of medical capability in 1800 (or even in 1868) that could not be made easily available outside the hospital's walls-at least in homes of the middle class and the wealthy. Physicians could ordinarily do little to alter the course of a patient's illness and almost as little to monitor quality of life on the ward. Contemporary therapeutics offered few procedures that could not be understood and evaluated by a well-in-formed layman. Much of household medicine was, in fact, identical with hospital treatment; indeed something of the social

---

[24] Rosenberg, Charles, E. The Care of Strangers, 1987, p. 4 -5

efficacy of early nineteenth-century therapeutics may *well have rested on this very community of* *understanding.* **The hospital in the early national** **America was defined primarily by need and** **dependency, not by the existence** *of* **specialized** **technical resources.**"[25]

The admission of the Hospital's first patient, Jacob Schwetzer typifies such a patient, chronically ill, indigent, needing chronic care, without hope of receiving treatment that would make a difference in his illness. Thus the doors of the ten room Asylum for Israelites on Monument and Ann Streets were open in 1868 with the corner stone laid on June 25 (see picture of corner stone). Dr. Joshua I. Cohen, vice president of Hebrew Benevolent Society, called the project, *"our long contemplated work, the* *founding and establishing of an institution under* *the auspices of our Society, for the purpose of bring* *additional comfort to the sick, poor and needy or* *our people."*[26]

---

[25] Ibid, p. 5.

[26] Umansky, Paul, Manager, Community Relations, digest intended in part to help develop material for Sinai" 124th anniversary in 1991 and to serve as a quick reference to events from the hospital's beginning to mid 1990. p.1

Record Book of the Hebrew Hospital and Asylum Association 1868 - 1877[27]

A review of the Record Book of the Hebrew Hospital and Asylum Association for the years 1868 through 1877, a large heavy leather bound volume, containing 573 pages, handwritten by the secretary, gives some flavor from the administrative viewpoint of the early history of the hospital. While the handwriting is in ink on remarkably well preserved paper, time and vicissitudes have made reading the script a challenge. The initial meeting was held on January 12, 1868 at the Metropolitan Hall in Baltimore. Jacob I. Cohen called the meeting to order and there proceeded with setting up Bylaws including Charter of the Association, Election of Board of Directors, Act of Corporation, Rules of Order, etc. "Any Israelite shall be admitted to the Hospital provided the resident or visiting Physician considers him in deed of medical treatment." Excluded were "applicants afflicted with a consanguineous or infectious Disease." A room was to be set aside for religious services.

The position of Steward is carefully delineated: "He shall be the Superintendent- carry out Board of Directors and Committees directives, keep a record of accounts and all monies received and disbursed, visit every ward at least once a day and before retiring, assure that nurses are at their posts and lights and fires in proper condition and door on premises securely fastened. He shall take particular

---

[27] Record Book of the Hebrew Hospital and Asylum Association, 1868-1877 Vol 1 was on exhibit in the glass case in the area of the hospital outside the dinning room. The case was kindly opened and I was given permission to review its contents.

care that no wine or spirits are used in the Hospital or Asylum except by Direction of the Physician for the use of the inmates." The duties of the Steward are further delineated. On the death of an Inmate the President is to be notified immediately and plans for disposal of the body arranged by friends or relations."

If an officer or person employed in the Hospital or Asylum shall use profane language.... (the rest was not legible).

The Board of Directors were diligent in their duties especially in addressing the financial condition of the new hospital. They were authorized to raise funds of $13,000 as noted in the secretary's report of 3/8/68 by issuing Certificates of Stock at $25 per share paying interest at 6% for 2 years. They carefully accounted for the bills including for coal $50, gas $12, wood $1.50, wine and liquor $10.00, work on cellar $4.00 and medicine for the Dispensary $10.00. Equally important was recording sources of income such as in the 4/4/69 meeting, Proceeds of the Purim Ball for furniture and bedding for Hospital, $1294.00

Beginning in the 4/3/1870 report was listing of admissions for the month: The amount the patient contributed is listed and if no listing the patient was free of any contribution, such as Sadie Cohen on March 1, 1870.

       Admissions
March 1   Sadie Cohen
March 21 Mrs Donasca $5.00/week
March 31 Spencer Ilafond $4.00/week
April 1   Rebecca Schafer $4.00/week

Discharges
March 5 Isadore Miller
March 8 John Rich

Deaths
March 3 James Atans

There is no listing of diagnosis or condition at discharge, this being primarily an administrative report. While the activity of admissions and discharges was rather limited initially the pace increases with time.

The meeting of 6/12/70 records the effort "to purchase 50 tons of hard coal and 15 tons of soft coal for the hospital at the cheapest price." Also at this meeting "A motion was resolved that a Committee shall be appointed to make arrangements for the erection of a dead house within the enclosure of the Hospital. (a dead house is probably a facility for autopsy) Bills for flowers and mattresses are recorded as well as the salary of the Steward/Superintendent for $281.57/month as well as that of the Secretary, $65.00 (a rather plush amount)

Report of monies received   in report of 7/3/70 include, "The treasurer's report that he received from the manager of the late Strawberry festival the sum of $1500." This was balanced by listing of bills to be paid, "work a the Hospital $100, gas bill $12.31, Ehrman Bros. for coal $105, Refreshments after meeting $9.80, Ice box $300, and the Steward's monthly salary of $298.71, and increase from $281.57, probably for excellent service.

Carrying out their supervisory function the report of 7/3/70 noted, "The Secretary was instructed to address the following note to the Attending Physician, Dr. Arnold, The note admonished Dr. Arnold requesting him politely "to be in the future more prompt on visiting the Institution and should he have professional or other engagements that prevent him from attending, to inform the President at his earliest convenience."

On the other hand the report of 8/8/70 indicates increase activity in the Hospital, "Letter to Hattie E. Allstone who wishes to be admitted to the Hospital. The Secretary was instructed to notify the lady that owing to the crowed state in the wards they are not able to admit her at present."

The transcript of the 3/5/71 meeting includes the following statement," It being stated that Lieberman (a patient in the Hospital)is a non paying inmate of the Asylum for the last two years who has a wealthy brother living in the City of London England. The Secretary was instructed to write to him to state the affairs of his brother and request him to compensate the Association." There is no follow up report on the success of this plan to secure payment for Lieberman's Asylum care.

An additional entry of 11/5/71 noted seven discharges and five admissions, three of whom paid $3-5/week. Committee on Purchase of grounds in rear of the Hospital also reported progress. A letter was directed to the Ladies of the Hebrews Hospital Association : *"Heart felt thanks for their untiring efforts and great zeal toward relocating and comforting the inmates of the Hebrew Hospital and Asylum. It would be impossible and an impossible loss to the Institution if the President and Managers of the Hebrew Hospital Association if the Ladies would cease to lend their helping hands. We therefore earnestly appeal to them to go on with their charitable and noble mission."* (This is the first report of friction between the Ladies Association and the Hospital)

Summary from the Record Book of the Hebrew Hospital and Association

The members of the Board of Directors of the Hebrew Hospital and Asylum Association met frequently and took their supervisory tasks seriously. They paid careful attention to the fiscal state of the new institution, attempted to obtain funds for its operation, detailed bills to be paid, carefully noting admissions, discharges and deaths without attention to diagnoses, length of stay or condition on discharge performing an administrative function. They took gentle disciplinary function on occasion and paid the secretary well and increased salary of the Superintendent as conditions indicated.

Summary of Highlights of Events through 1900

1870-1879 In this decade the hospital is overcrowded. There is not enough funding, not enough trained nurse; doctors complain. According to the log, there are many applicants for the position of steward, mostly men who were unsuccessful in business. Hospital directors select those whose wives are good cooks!

One of the directors "unjustly criticized the Ladies Auxiliary for "not contributing any important aid to the Hospital." The women could not be placated after this accusation and the group disbanded. (This rift would be not be repaired until 1948 that "the women of the community saw the need to reestablish their formal role as advocates for this growing and vital Jewish institution.)[28]

1880-1889 The city condemns Milliman Street (see map—a small street between Monument and Madison, that no longer exits) to let the hospital add a new a new building (in 1886) and renovate the old one. 1884   Colonel Benjamin E. Ulman serves a s president for one year. 1885 Mike Friedman served as president until his death in 1903) 1889 A "substantial apothecary" is established

b) A hospital dispensary area is added, and a dispensary service is open at all times as a free outpatient department.

c) New method is devised to prescribe and label medicine.

d) a new diet table and methods to prescribe suitable patient diets is created.

e) Operating room is rebuilt

f) A small new build houses the laundry and two wards for consumptive patients.

1890-1899 Lack of funds is a continuing problem. Problems continue in caring for chronic patients,

---

[28] Umansky, Paul, Story of Sinai Hospital 1866-1959, Reflections, a publication for the Jewish Museum of Maryland, July 1997, P8.

while trying to maintain facilities for the growing number of acutely ill.

1895 Report by the resident physician (a staff physician hired by the hospital), Dr. Melvin S. Rosenthal :

"...attention must be drawn to the improved character of work of our hospital. It has been our earnest endeavor to relieve acute suffering...and such cases as promise improvement by surgical medical aid, assisted by nourishment and hygienic surroundings were especially sought after. We point with pardonable pride to the number of children rescued from deformity and life of dependence. These case are a expense to the institution, but when we note the fact that ewe have relieved society from life-long objects of charity.. the end justifies the means."

An entire ward was devoted to treating children, separating them from the adult sick and aged.

Effort also is made to separate home for aged with hospital patients.

Consumptives are no longer accepted, in the belief that fresh air is more beneficial than hospital care. (Patients like Jacob Schwetzer would presumably no long be eligible for admission)

An era of "modern surgery" begins with construction of an up to date operating room."

So that by 1900 we have made slow but significance in changing The Asylum for the Israelites into a Hospital. There is now a modern operating room, a

Resident Physician, children are being separated from the adult sick and aged, no longer are tuberculosis patients being admitted but being farmed out to the then popular fresh air treatment plan, while nutrition, hygienic surroundings and relief of acute suffering remain the major therapeutic measures under the influence of Florence Nightingale and others.

However, "the emphasis (on care) was already shifting from maintenance of chronic patients to curing of acute illness."[29] Dr. Eugene J. Leopold recalls, " That the hospital was growing, is evinced by the fact that an addition was built on the rear of the original building, which about doubled the capacity of the Hospital. This permitted a temporary separation of the sick and the Aged... Well do I recall, the cow shed with its two cows located a short distance south of the building. Next to the cow shed was a wooden shack, which housed several patients with 'consumption.'"[30]

While one of the purposes of the establishment of a Jewish Hospital was to provide a placed for Jewish physicians to practice medicine, according to Paul Umansky, "Dr. A.D. Stein was appointed the first resident physician to attend patients (and) by 1889 there were six doctors on the staff, most of them non-Jewish because of the scarcity of Jewish physicians."[31]

[29] Shapiro, M. Sigmund, Sinai Hospital of Baltimore,Inc. Centennial Anniverary Paper, 5/8/1966, p. 3.

[30] Leopold, Eugene J. M.D. , History of Sinai Hospital, School of Nursing Announcement, 1943, p. 4.

[31] Umansky, Paul, Story of Sinai Hospital 1866 – 1959, July 1997, p.3.

Influence of the Opening of the Johns Hopkins Hospital across the Street in 1893

The big elephant just across the street, The Johns Hopkins Hospital with its emphasis on scholarship, research and clinical medicine had opened its doors in 1893. William Osler had written his classic Text Book of Medicine in 1892 but I find no reference to any interchange, either referral of patients or consultation of any of the "Big Four" to its neighbor just across the street. This relationship too would require a number of years to develop.

But the Asylum for the Israelites was making progress so that by 1900 the shift from custodial care of the poor and ill was being morphed into the modern concept of a hospital. The era of making a therapeutic difference with medications and surgery had not as yet arrived but was on the horizon.

Making of the Asylum for Israelites into Sinai Hospital 1900 – 1959

What can be expected from the next sixty years as the Asylum for the Israelites converts itself into Sinai Hospital? Thirty four patients were treated in the initial year of operation, 1868, by 1902 the Hospital had treated 396 patients in the year 1902.[32] These are some of the major events of the years 1900 -1960 which would include: [33]

---

[32] Leopold, Eugene J. , History of Sinai Hospital, 1943 p.4.

[33] Umansky, Paul, History of Sinai Hospital of Baltimore, 125th Anniversary Highlights of Events by Decade, 1863-199,. 1991

1. Additional facilities and buildings would be on the horizon.

2, Nursing School was opened in 1906,

3. A patient with typhoid fever was admitted 1911. This is a summary of a detailed report of this patient, Ezra Jones, at the Hebrew Hospital and Asylum. He was admitted with a temperature of 104 degrees on April 19th, 1911 and remained above 100 degrees with spikes to above 104 for forty one days until 5/30/11 before being discharged, "cured" on June 20th. He was 33 years old and lived at 20 E. Franklin Street and worked as a manager of a light company. He complained of headaches, chills and fever. The initial diagnostic impression is left blank. A detailed history and physical examination in fairly legible handwriting is recorded by Dr. McCall. There were no localizing signs and abdomen while full was soft and *one suspicious rose spot* was noted. Progress note of 4/21/11 reported *two suspicious rose spots.* Intermittent episodes of delirium were recorded in the progress notes that extended to 6/28/11. While the physician's notes are minimal the record is replete in carefully handwritten legible notes from the nursing staff. Temperature is recorded six to eight times per day, medications are carefully listed Arom. Spt. of Am. (Aromatic spirits of ammonia), Urotropin, whisky, morphine on occasion, Strycn/ Tr. Nux Vom (Strychnine/Tincture of Nux vomia) as a stimulant, etc. Nurses report on his mental and physical state, noting at times delirium, confused, state of appetite, etc. Lab test are sparse but include a urinalysis: two plus albumin, rbcs, few wbc an amorphous urates, Wbc 8,400 and a *positive Widal test* on 4/24/11 (Gruber –Widal

test for typhoid fever: to dilutions of patients serum are added equal volume of dilutions with 24 hr. bouillon culture of Salmonella typhosa looking for flocculations and precipitation for a positive test) Mr. Ezra Jones was afebrile from the forty first day through 70th day on June 20th. Discharge summary is brief: *Patient entered hospital complaining of headache, chills and fever. Under treatment outlined above patient improved and left hospital on June 28, '11, Cured. Diagnosis: Typhoid*

My summary: Two rose spots and a positive Widal test with fever with delirium for forty days and total hospital stay of 70 days.

4. Chiefs of Service were designated by 1920 – Dr. B. Bernheim in Surgery, Dr. Charles Austrian in Medicine, Dr. M. Aaronson in Obstetrics and Dr. Eugene J. Leopold as Chairman of the Medical Board ,

5. Change of the name of Hebrew Hospital to Sinai Hospital of Baltimore was made in 1926, and surgery becomes fully approved by the American Surgical Association

6. Hospital gains AMA approval to train interns and residents.in 1928.

7. Tobias Weinberg in 1939 become first full-time Pathologist in Chief.

8. Harvey Weiss becomes Executive Director. I knew him and his family well and were neighbors in the late 1940ies.

9. The establishment of a department of research both in pathology and Urology, The Hoffberger Urological Research Center in 1940 under Drs Goldstein and Abeshouse.

10. The E.M. Bluestone report of 1944 recommending move of the Sinai Hospital from its location on Monument Street, then for 76 years, to northwest Baltimore, the site of migration of the Jewish population, combining the already established Levindale Chronic Hospital with Mount Pleasant Hospital for tuberculosis then located west of Reisterstown. This move would be accomplished sixteen years later in 1960, initiating a new and expanded hospital. (See below for a discussion of the Bluestone report)

11. Reestablishment of the Sinai Auxiliary in 1948, after criticism of the Ladies Auxiliary in the 1870ies for " not contributing any important aid to the hospital." According to the report of Paul Umansky the Auxiliary organized the first children's play room, brought books to patients, established a gift shop and canteen.[34]

12. Establishment of full time department heads first in Radiology 1950, Dr. Julian O. Salik, Pediatrics 1953, Dr. Harry Gordon, Surgery 1954, Dr. Arnold Seligman and Dr. Albert Mendeloff in

---

[34] Umansky, Paul, Reflections, a publication of the Jewish Museum of Maryland, p. 8-9.

Medicine 1955, [35] all with joint appointment s with Johns Hopkins and beginning of interexchange of house staff and activities with Hopkins.

13. Among many new programs was the initiation of hemodilaysis in 1957 using a twin coil Travenol artificial kidney, originally developed by Willhem Kolph in the Netherlands during World War 11. Sinai's use of this early model of the twin coil kidney was its second employment in Baltimore, following that at the Baltimore City Hospital.

14. The year before the move from the old Monument Street location to Greespring and Belevdere Avenues, the Sinai Hospital Journal recorded a list of Publications just for the period January 1, 1959 among the staff of Sinai Hospital. This is truly a remarkable list of publications indicating the volume and breath of activities from the clinical and laboratory investigation that emanated form a relative small hospital primarily

---

[35] I knew Drs. Mendeloff and Seligman very well. Dr. Mendeloff and I first became acquainted with while an Intern and Assistant Resident at Barnes Hospital in St. Louis in 1953-55 where he was a GI consultant and worked in this lab. He had been trained at the Mass Memorial Hospital in Boston under Dr. Ingelfinger. After he was appointed as chief of Medicine in 1955, I became chief resident at Sinai in 1958-59. Following that I shared a neighboring office for many years. His interests were protean but I especially enjoyed his knowledge of music. Dr. Seligman had been trained at Beth Israel in Boston and was a first rate biochemist and continued his interest in this field while at Sinai. I remember him especially for his interest and knowledge in fishing. He stocked a pond on his property with fish from New England and I had the pleasure of accompanying my son on one occasion to his pond where we caught two fish on two prepared hooks simultaneously, a feat never before or after experienced by me. Dr. Seligman then demonstrated his skill at surgery by filleting the fish on the spot.

devoted to clinical care. I have taken the liberty to list only some of these reports so that the number and variety of investigations can be appreciated:

a. Abeshouse, G.A., Goldstein, R. B., and Abeshouse B.S. Adrenal Cysts reported in J. of Urology, 81:711, 1959   The Hoffberger Urological Research Lab under Drs. Abeshouse and Goldstein provided a fertile and productive activity

b. Bix, Harold and Marriott, Henry: Reciprocal Beats Masquerading as Ventricular Captures. AM. J. of Cardiology 4: 128, 1959. Harold Bix was a cardiologist from Vienna with a vast knowledge of information in the field of EKG.

c. Blumenfeld, H.L. and Rogers D.E. Studies of Influenza, J. Clin.Invest, 38:199, 1959. Dr. Herbert Blumenfeld did this work while a fellow in Infectious Disease at Cornell with Dr. Rogers. He became Chief Resident in Medicine at Sinai

d. Conn, Jacob: On the History of Hypnosis. Instit. For Res in Hypnosis 1959. Dr. Conn was a psychiatrist in practice at Hopkins and Sinai who has five additional reports in this list of publications.

e. Cornblath, M. et al : Symptomatic Neonatal Hypoglycemia. M. Pediat., 55: 545,   1959. Dr. Cornblath was in the Depart of Pediatics and later became Professor and head of Dept of Pediatics at the University of Maryland.

f. Gordon, H.H. and Nitowsky, H. M. Vitamin E, Modern Nutrition in Health and Disease, 1959. He became Professor of Pediatics at Albert Einstein College of Medicine.

g. Hoffman, E.: Peptic ulcer in Massive Hemorrhage, J. Am. Geriatics Soc. 4 324, 1958. Dr. Hoffman was trained at Hopkins and was active on surgical service at Sinai. H contributed six additional papers in this year on a variety of topics.

h. Mendeloff, A.I.: Chapter 19 "Constipation and Diarrhea" in Harrison Text Book of Medicine, 1958. Dr. Mendeloff was chief of the medical service for 25 years beginning in 1957.

i. Nachlas, M.M.: A Critical Evaluatin of Colorimetirc Determination of Urinary Lipase, J. Bio. Chem. 230:1051, 1959. Dr. Nachlas was in the Dept of Surgery and published papers with Dr. Seligman as well as clinical papers on Surgery. He contributed an additional seven papers to this list of publications in 1958.

j. Seligman,A.M. Contributed ten papers with a variety of authors on biochemical and tumor related subjects.

This is only a partial list of the Publications listed in the Sinai Hospital Journal for the year 1958 and included an additional 150 papers. A similar list of publication for the year Jan. 1958-Dec. 1958 includes many of these same authors including Levy, R.I., Weiner, I.M. , Mudge, G.H., JCI 37,146, 1958, Effect of Acid Base Balance on the Diuresis produced by Organic and Inorganic Mercurals,

Expansion of Facilities with Addition of New Buildings

The Frank building was erected in 1906 by the gift of $80,000 from the widow of Dr. Samuel Leon Frank who had been a former hospital president. This allowed for the separation of the hospital from the Home for the Aged as well as private rooms and allowed the more affluent in the population to consider a hospital rather than care at home. On the top floor were two modern operating rooms and out patient facilities in the basement. A Training School for Nurses was built in 1907, followed by the Hecht Nursing Home for student nurses in 1912 and the Mendels Maternity Building and Hess Dispensary in 1915.

Samuel Schmidt was a physician at Mercy Hospital who was friendly with Dr. Alfred Ulman,[36] head of surgical department at Sinai, and at Dr. Schmidt's death in 1917 he left $300,000 and combined with gifts from additional donors and with the help of the Associated Jewish Charities additional funds for the construction of a seven story building which opened in 1927 giving the hospital 220 beds.

The Bluestone Report: A study of the Medical Activities of the 'associated Jewish Charities, Baltimore, Maryland by E.M. Bluestone, M.D.

This report of E. M. Bluestone in 1944 was probably the most significant event in the sixty years under consideration, 1900-1960 for the Sinai Hospital of Baltimore.

---

[36] Dr. Alfred Ulman has a special relationship with me in that in 1934 he performed an appendectomy on me at the Sinai Hospital.

This report of E. M. Bluestone, who was a physician and director of the Montefiore Hospital in New York since 1934. His bibliography includes many articles on Medical care of the aged, Hospitals for chronic disease, and Planning for long-term care. As the title of the report would indicates the report was authorized by the Associated Jewish Charities of Baltimore.[37] In Bluestones introductory letter to Milton E. Gundersheimer, Acting Executive Director of the AJC, Bluestone indicates, "You asked me for an over-all statement and a plan for the future development of you medical institution." The report is a ninety six page in depth evaluation of "your medical activities in addition to a constructive plan for their future." Bluestone recognized, "the intelligence and philanthropic spirit of your community are beyond praise." He goes on to indicated that, "Your may assume that I have examined every scrap of evidence that has a bearing on the problem and that my conclusions were unhurried and carefully weighed....I earnestly hope that these conclusions will fascinate you as they have fascinate this student of the hospital scene." Most cogent is Bluestones method of approach:

*My method of approach to the Baltimore problem was somewhat **clinical in nature**. The preventive aspects of*

---

[37] The Associated Jewish Charities was formed in 1920 from the amalgamation of 13 agencies which composed the Federated Jewish Charities (organized in 1906) and the nine agencies which made up the United Hebrew Charities (organized in 1909). Earlier organization included the Hebrew Benevolent Society founded in 1854 which was instrumental in helping founding the Hebrew Hospital and Asylum in 1863, as noted above under the topic of Early History o f the Sinai Hospital of Baltimore.

*medical service were always before me and I did, indeed ,
face the Baltimore situation with the question in my
mind as to how similar shortcomings can be prevented
from recurring. I examined the signs and symptoms in
order to establish a diagnosis, and in this respect I was
aided by valuable laboratory assistance. The cure
recommended is based on successful experimental data
and on opinion which is rapidly crystallizing in to
unanimity. The patient* (ie the hospital) *with whom I
dealt was a composite patient, who must be seen in a
total way, and dealt with as a total personality by total
methods.*

Bluestone indicates in his first twenty pages of
introduction that for his report and evaluation of
the current situation of Sinai Hospital on
Monument Street he "interviewed most of the key
medical officers, as well as the administrative
executives as well as the visiting staff,
Commissioner of Health, deans of Johns Hopkins
and University of Maryland, director of the
Hopkins Hospital, director of Blue Cross plan of
Baltimore, prominent members of the Jewish
medical community including Mr. Hutzler and Dr.
Austrian." His purpose was to obtain "a frank
appraisal of your medical activities, in addition to a
constructive plan for their future." He commented
that "the intelligence and philanthropic spirit of
your community are beyond praise." He indicated
that "You may assume that I have examined every
scrap of evidence that has a bearing on the problem
and that my conclusions were unhurried and
carefully weighed."

There then follows a discussion of "medical care in
a changing world...and hospital history being
rewritten under the stimulus of the profound social

change..." He discusses the change in treatment of tuberculosis from emphasizing change in climate, rest and fresh air to more active treatment... (Streptomycin had been just introduced as treatment for tuberculosis). The true medical center is the one which studies the natural history of disease in all of its phases, from infancy to old age, in a group of buildings which may be physically set apart, but which are integrated under a single medical social plan." Rather than speaking of "chronic" care the term "long-term care" is being considered. Dr. Bluestone in his report seemed very interested in long term care, "It is in the field of long –term medicine that the scientist finds his greatest opportunity." Integration of in-patient and out patient departments was discussed. He emphasized the need for a full time medical directors, adequate laboratory space, need for a home care program, a rehabilitation program and the need to eliminate open wards.

Following this introduction the Bluestone reports examines the deficits in the current situation of Sinai Hospital. The absence of any provision for "Negro" care was noted, the need to support education and research, the establishment of a social service department and a woman's auxiliary inadequate power plant, laundry, cafeteria. He noted the need for a senior medical officer in each of the specialties, as well as the need for graduate medical education. He emphasized the need for Rehabilitation and Home Care facilities. On item he felt was not necessary was the establishment of a Medical School.

Bluestone's major recommendation was a move of the hospital from the East Baltimore location to

Northwest Baltimore where the Jewish population had already migrated, since there was no hospital facility at that time in this area.[38] The major point was to combine the facilities of the tuberculosis hospital, Mt. Pleasant then located west of Resisterstown in the open country, as had been the prevailing opinion for care of tuberculosis before antibiotics, with the already established chronic care facility of Levindale in NW Baltimore. This would necessitate the moving the inadequate facilities of the Monument Street location of Sinai, combining these facilities into one major hospital center.

Levindale had been established in 1921, initially to combine two orphan asylums, one in the slums of East Baltimore and the other in west Baltimore on the site of what was to become the old West Baltimore Hospital[39]. "Levindale" was named after Louis H. Levin, the first director of the Associated Jewish Charities. The plan for Levindale became obsolete when the The White House Conference held during the presidency of William H. Taft recommended foster homes instead of institutions for such children and with the overcrowding of the Hebrew Home for the Aged and Infirm and the adjacent Hebrew Friendly Inn on Aisquith Street in East Baltimore became badly overcrowded and required renovation, Levindale became an instant

---

[38] Interestingly, Montefiore Hospital where Bluestone was Director of the Hospital, had originally been a chronic facility for invalids and chronically ill, much as the original Asylum for Israelites had been, but in 1912 in "search for open spaces" had moved to the Bronx for just such reasons as Bluestone was suggesting for Sinai's move.

[39] The title Hebrew Orphan Asylum still is engraved on the red brick building on Rayner Avenue in West Baltimore.

alternative solution. At the time the location of Levindale , "being out in the wilds", was a concern but the institution developed into a model geriatric care center. It was this amalgamation of facilities, bringing Mt. Pleasant in from the country and Sinai Hospital out of East Baltimore on to the area of the already established Levindale that was the heart of the Bluestone report.

Bluestone had specific recommendation for the organization and architectural plans for the new hospital. His one negative caveat was "no capital funds will be sunk into such projects as gymnasium or a swimming pool." However he was very specific in recommending, "In such a center as I have in mind for you, we shall need the highest type of scientist and hospital worker. Every organizational move that is made hence forth from the board of trustees down, should be activated by the necessity for acquiring the best in every field. Suggestions for fund raising and avoidance of a mortgage were noted. The development of a Joint Administrative Board for problems of financing, community relationships, fundamental policy, research and education program was suggested. He argued "against any ward unit. Rather than wards he recommended adequate provision for one and two-bed units to provide easy nursing supervision." Detailed architectural plans were promulgated:

So far as the height is concerned," *I believe that you will require ten stories in the central building* (only five were built for the original building but plans for seven were made), *with executive offices placed on the ground floor. It will, I believe, be of considerable importance for the architects to plan a foundation for each of the buildings that will be strong enough to sustain additional stories if they should be required with the passage of time.* (You can see that he was from New York)

Bluestone recommended a building for the study of pulmonary diseases as well as a building for long-term care both of which was never accomplished However his suggestions for an out-patient building of three floors as well as an auditorium were accepted and eventually a psychiatric building was built. He even discussed a central power plant, laundry, kitchens and employees' dining rooms   but left their   location   to the consulting engineers.

Dr. Bluestones' concept of abandoning the East Baltimore Monument Street location of Sinai Hospital and combining the already existant Mt. Pleasant on the site of Levindale in Northwest Baltimore was the core of the plan.[40] Much of the plan was effectuated as Bluestone proposed : the general lay out of the hospital, avoiding wards, administration offices on the first floor, out patient building of three floors, and psychiatric building that was added later. He didn't anticipate the research building that was provided by Ancel Schonenman but a pulmonary building was never

------

[40] "Mount Pleasant, a tuberculosis facility moved in 1952 from Reisterstown to Sinai's current location in preparation of the unification. It became part of Sinai after the hospital arrived in 1959. Sinai and Levindale only exchanged patients and physicians as the need arose. It wasn't until July 1, 1996, that the institutions finally merged as Sinai Health System. I took 37 years, and the impetus was born of the need for foth to prosper in the current health care climate."   Umansky, Paul, Story of Sinai Hospital 1866-1959, in Reflections, a publication of the Jewish Museum of Maryland, July 1997, p. 11.

built. Included was also the warning that was followed, *"I earnestly hope that no capital funds will be sunk into such projects as a gymnasium or swimming pool in either of these buildings."* (much to the disappointment of successive house staff appointments. The Johns Hopkins eventually did provide these very same amenities for their facility.)

There is no discussion of the down side of this plan with respect to the negative aspect of being removed from the immediate vicinity of Johns Hopkins Hospital and the easy liaisons and ease of sharing medical consultation and activities to complement a smaller hospital. After leaving East Baltimore, Hopkins promptly bought the land and facilities that eventually became their Turner Auditorium, leaving not a trace of the old Hebrew Hospital.

The inability to upgrade or expand the facilities in East Baltimore and the opportunity to centralize medical care in the area to which the Jewish population had moved, establishing a medical center combining Mt. Pleasant and Levindale, had seemed to trump the concept of not moving, even if it would lose the easy access to Hopkins presence. The Bluestone plan in much of its detail was accepted and effectuated by the move to present facilities in 1959 after adequate funding, fifteen years after in was promulgated.

Move to the new facilities at Belvedere and
Greenspring Avenues
1959 through 2009

According to Mr. Paul Umansky the move from the old hospital on Monument Street to its present location at Belvedere and Greenspring Avenues was " one the smoothest logistical maneuvers one could wish for."[41] I can attest to this opinion being a recently appointed Attending Physician and accompanying the caravan that resulted in the transfer. About a dozen ambulances were assembled to transport the ill patients that could not be transported otherwise or discharged and a long line of cars and vans transported the reduced census of patients that could not be discharge. The patients and staff followed finding an elegant, spick and span facility much modernized from that on Monument Street. Mount Pleasant which had already moved to the new location was intergrated into the new hospital and the second floor initially was used as the site for the service patients, all rooms being private or semi private rooms as suggested by the Bluestone report. The first floor of the Mt. Pleasant Building provided an area for inpatient psychiatric patients. The suggestion of Bluestone for an expanded pulmonary service for the Mt Pleasant Building in this case was not fulfilled.

The One Hundredth Year of Sinai Hospital 1966

The Sinai Hospital Journal recorded a symposium, June 11 and 12 on the Centennial Celebration of Sinai Hospital. Included on this occasion was a biographical digest and appreciation of Drs. Milton Sherry and Albert Goldstein who had died that year as well as by Dr. B.S. Abeshouse, chief of Urology. Additional papers included talks by Dr. Sol Sherry, Professor of Medicine at Washington

---

[41] Umansky, Paul, Story of Sinai Hospital 1866-1959, Reflections, p.12.

University School of Medicine, Dr. Paul H. Lavietes from Yale, Dr. Bernard Tabatznik head of Cardiology at Sinai, Dr. Ivan L. Bennett, Jr, Pathologist-in-Chief at Johns Hopkins, Dr. Leonard Scherlis, head of Cardiology at U. of Maryland, as well as Drs. Harry Gordon, Milton Markowitz, Frank F. Furstenberg, Dr. A. M. Seligman, Chief of Surgery at Sinai and many others.

Additions and Expansion of Services at Sinai in Northwest Baltimore

Following the move to the "New " Sinai Hospital in 1959 there were a steady and increasing array of increasing programs and activities stimulated by this move.

The Department of Psychiatry was established with an out patient Rymland Building to be built next to Mt. Pleasant and a further out patient building in the years to come. In the 1970ies a coronary care unit was established as well as an expanded ICU on the fourth floor of the main building. A sixth floor for 51 private patient rooms was added to the original five floors of the new Sinai Hospital, approaching the seven floors recommended by the Bluestone report.

In the 1970ies an enlarged 21 bed ICU on the fourth floor of the Hospital was established.

In the 1980ies Drs. Michael Mirowski and Morton Mower developed the Automatic Implantable Cardiac Defibrillator, developed at Sinai in the basement of the Shapiro Research Building and clinically applied to a patient at Hopkins.[42] The device has been universally accepted to treat cardiac arrest by the implanted device being able to recognize an arrhythmia and provide an electrical stimulation to revert the arrhythemia. A fitting memorial plaque is now in the lobby of the hospital. The site of this original and probably the most important research achievement of Sinai Hospital to date was performed in the basement of this Shapiro Research Building, a facility not envisaged or proposed by the Bluestone Report.

In patient Homodialysis Unit was also established.

Ansel and Ellen Schoeneman donation helped with the building of a beautiful building in the front of the Hospital for the new department of Rehabilitation Medicine under Dr. Cohen. A Traumatic Brain injury unit was established in Mt. Pleasant. Sinai Fitness established itself in Owings Mills. Dr. Richard Aach became Chief of Medicine with further integrated programs of medicine and surgery with Hopkins.

In the 1990s a Joint Center was established. There was increased emphasis on cancer chemotherapy. A new ER 7 was built as well.

---

[42] Dr. Mirowski, born in Poland, trained in France and had brief experience at Hopkins was recruited by Dr. Mendeloff to head up the Coronary Care Unit. He had had the idea of an automatic cardiac defibrillator for some time and with the help of Dr. Mower who had been a house staff officer and Attending perfected the device in the dog lab of the Schoenman Research Building. My contribution to Dr. Mirowski's introduction to America was my detailed explanation of his queers about baseball.

In the 2000s The Rubin Institute for Advanced Orthopedics was established with a new four story building on top of the Rehabilitation Building. The Spine Center at Sinai was opened in 2003 as well as a Sleep Center in the Shapiro Building as well as a Cyber Knife facility. In 2004 the Hackerman-Patz Guest House was erected to provide a location for over night stays for visitors to the Hospital. A Brain and Spine Unit offering a full range of services combining neurosurgery, neurology, orthopedics, rebab and physical medicine is established. Sinai Hospital morphs itself into a new entity, LifeBridge Health, combining a myriad of activities and organization, Sinai Hospital, North West Hospital, Levindale, LifeBridge Gym, and various out patient clinics and related facilities. The beautiful large addition to the hospital has been a fitting expansion on its 50th anniversary of the move from Monument Street in 2009 with provisions for an expanded ICU and acute care facilities.

These are just a sampling of the growth and expansion of Sinai Hospital with wide ranging activities in the health care arena. As the Hospital approaches its 50th anniversary in its current location at Greenspring Ave. and Northern Pky and its 146th year anniversary since the founding of the Hospital in 1863 at Monument and Ann Streets there has been tremendous development and progress. The Bluestone report of 1944 charted the way for an independent Jewish facility, removed from the enveloping influence of the neighboring behemoth, the Johns Hopkins Hospital, and set Sinai Hospital on a path to establish its own Center of influence. What would have been the result of Sinai Hospital remaining adjacent to Hopkins, becoming affiliated with it and becoming a joint entity with Hopkins, much as the Jewish Hospital and Barnes Hospital in St Louis or the Beth Israel with the Harvard Hospitals in Boston? The progressive logarithmic development of Sinai Hospital in its new location has provided an independent facility with multiple arms of activities that rivals independent Jewish Hospitals in other cities arguing favorably for the move from East Baltimore. From the Hebrew Hospital and Asylum in 1863 (aka Israelite Asylum) to the Sinai Hospital in 1926, in East Baltimore at the corner of Monument and Ann Streets(Rutland Ave) and then to its transformation to its current location at Northern Parkway and Greenspring Ave and morphing itself under the banner of LifeBridge Health with many related activities in 2000 in the health care field has been an accelerating and stimulating adventure in bringing health care and related activities to Northwest Baltimore.

Chapter Two

Sir William Osler's View on Pierre C.A. Louis' Recommendations for Bleeding In Pneumonia—Paradox of Calling his Method Iconoclastic Continuing Practice of Bleeding

"La Barriere contre l'esprit du systeme"[1]
"Medicina est ars conjecturalis"[2]
"There are many stars in Paris, but Louis is the sun"[3]

---

[1] Pierre Louis wrote to his Boston disciple Henry I. Bowditch, reminding him of the duty they both had embraced to stand stalwart, as Louis put it, at *"la Barriere contre l'espirit du systeme" (the Barricade against the spirit of the system)* as quoted by John Harley Warner in his book by the same name, Against the Spirit of the System – The French impulse in Nineteenth Century American Medicine, Princeton University Press, p. 5, 1998.

[2] "Medicine is an art based on inconclusive or incomplete evidence" as quoted by Willliam August Guy as the opening statement in his article *On the Value of the Numerical Method as Applied to Science, but Especially to Physiology and Medicine,* Journal of the Statistical Society of London, Vol; 2. No 1, (Feb, 1839) pp. 25.

[3] Memoirs of Marshall Hall by his widow, Charlotte Hall, London, 1861, p, 194. "He (Marshall Hall) became as it were, again a pupil accompanying M. Louis in his early clinical visits at the hospital, admiring his acumen and careful diagnosis. 'There are many stars in Paris, but Louis is the sun', he as been heard to say."

Objectives

1. Review of background leading to Pierre Louis'questioning of bleeding in pneumonia

2. Evaluate Louis' *methode numerique* with emphasis on careful observation and enumeration of results

3. Explain William Osler's admiration of Pierre Louis, including his Essay on *The Influence of Louis on American Medicine* and visiting his tomb, yet his continuing recommendations for bleeding in pneumonia in spite of Louis' studies showing the "narrow limits to the utility of this mode of treatment."

In the third edition of William Osler's Principles and Practice of Medicine, 1897, regarding recommendations for bleeding in pneumonia, are the lines:

"The reproach of van Helmont that a bloody Molock presides in the chairs of medicine[4] cannot be brought against the present generation of physicians.

Before Louis' iconoclastic paper on bleeding in pneumonia it would have been considered almost criminal to treat a case without venesection.

During the first five decades of the century the profession bled too much, but during the last decade we have certainly bled too little. Pneumonia is one of the diseases in which a timely venesection may save lives. <u>To be of service it should be done early</u>"

Pierre Louis' paper, *Researches on the Effect of Bloodletting in some Inflammatory Disease*,[5] published in 1828 called into question the value of

---

[4] Thanks to the personal communication of Professor IML Donaldson of the University of Edinburgh I have learned that "a bloody Moloch presides in the chair of medicine" appears in the *Oriatrike* of Van Helmont, Ortus medicinae, Amsterdam, 1648, chapter 56, Pleura furens; section 34, next to last sentence in the paragraph, *"At certecruentum Molik, Cathedris Praesidere conspicuo medicis.* (On the other hand undoubtedly, I observe a bloody moloch to preside in the Chairs of medicine, translated by John Chandler, 1662.) Interestingly the reference is not a plea for the abolishment of bleeding, which however Van Helmont was very much in favor, but as a reaction to the excessive use of clysters (enemas) in the management of GI bleed. He felt that blood in the gut was not harmful, "the natural tear doth not bite the Eye thereof, neither the Urine the Bladder. So also the Dung in a Bowel... which is natural excrement. But that a Clyster doth pain, because it is a foreigner to a Bowel.

[5] Louis, Pierre, Ch.A., Reasearches on the Effects of Bloodletting in some Inflammatory Diseases, Archives Generales de Medecine.Memoires and Observations, November 1828, p. 322-336.

phlebotomy in pneumonia. How then could William Osler call Louis' paper iconoclastic and in the same breath recommend that bleeding should be performed more frequently and early as well? Textbooks contemporaneous with Osler's *Principles and Practice of Medicine* by Alfred Loomis and Austin Flint had found little to recommend bleeding in pneumonia at the end of the 19th century.[6] Oliver Wendell Holmes in his farewell address at the Harvard Medical School in 1882 referred to bloodletting as a past "wonder-worker in disease now thankfully discarded."[7]

William Olser was an admirer of Pierre Louis and praised him in the essay on *The Influence of Louis on American Medicine* [8] as well as visiting his grave in Paris in 1905. Osler in this paper on Louis quotes correctly Louis's conclusions, 1. "pneumonia is never arrested at once by blood letting" and 2. "the supposed happy effects on the progress of the disease were very much less than was commonly

---

[6] Loomis, Alfred, Textbook of Practical Medicine 5th edition, p. 123 and Flint Austin, A Treatise on the Principles and Practice of Medicine, 1894, p.86-87. Flint states, "Experience has already shown that (bleeding) cannot be relied upon to arrest this (condition). The probability of success is not sufficient to warrant its employment."

[7] Holmes, Oliver Wendell , Medical essays 1843-1882 (Boston, 1888), p.432. Holmes continues, "The lancet was the magician's wand of the dark ages of medicine." This address also contains Homes reminiscences on his contact with P. Louis in Paris in 1930.

[8] Osler, William, The Influence of Louis on American Medicine, Read before the Stille Society of the Medical Department of the University of Pennsylvania. Reprinted in The Johns Hopkins Hospital Bulletin Nos 77-78 August-September 1897. Reprinted in Alabama Student and other biographical essays, 1908

believed." Recognizing these conclusions why did Osler not follow Louis' advice and temper his use of blood letting in pneumonia? Why the enthusiasm of Osler for bleeding in pneumonia? Did Osler have an alternative interpretation of the results of Louis, or did he consider that the data were not entirely convincing? Could there have been other reasons for his position which was against the grain of prevailing medical opinion at the time? These are the questions to be considered in this paper.

Louis' Method

Louis' method was to gather together a sufficient number of cases of a similar condition and tabulate them so that the results of therapeutic maneuver could be evaluated. He stressed the importance of accurate observation, carefully describing the historical and clinical condition to be as certain as possible that the subjects all had a similar condition. He divided the patients into a group treated early and a group with similar diagnostic features treated later in the disease, noting time of onset and convalescence. Perhaps is was this empirical method and its careful execution that Osler could have considered *iconoclastic* in his paper rather than the interpretation or conclusion of the results.

Louis could find little difference between the effectiveness of early or late bleeding.

Osler in his essay on Louis, rather than focusing on Louis' methods and conclusions placed great emphasis on the influence of Louis on the many young American physicians such as James Jackson,

Jr., Henry I. Bowditch, Oliver Wendell Holmes etc, who went to Paris in the 1830's and brought back with them an approach to medicine mirroring that of their teacher. It was these Americans and other foreign students who studied with Louis who organized the Society of Medical Observation (*Societe Mediale d'Observation*) where frequent debates on theory and practice of medicine took place. Let us briefly review some of these debates as they set the stage for evaluating Louis' methods.

Debate at the Royal Academy of Medicine in Paris

An example of such a debate at the Royal Academy of Medicine in Paris was between M. Francois Double who argued for the "Inapplicability of Statistics to the Practice of Medicine" and Pierre Louis who supported the Application of Statistics to Medicine.[9] These debates translated into English with editorial comments were published in the *American Journal of the Medical Sciences*[10] in 1837,

---

[9] Rosen, George Problems in the Application of statistical analysis to Qestions of Health 1700-1880, Bulletin of the History of Medicine 29, p. 36, 1953. Rosen points out, "...in 1817, when the French Academy of Science proposed a prize to encourage statistical studies, *statistics* was defined as a "science of facts,"..."

[10] The American Journal of the Medical Sciences is the oldest medical journal in America founded in 1827. It was edited by Dr. Isasc Hayes for 52 years. Its format included original articles, review of recent medical publications, and periscope (abstracts) in medical progress in all parts of the world. *According to The Development of the Medical Science in the 19th Century* as recorded in the *American Journal of the Medical Science* in 1901, "it aided in developing and maintaining the influence of the French School of Medicine with American Physicians for many years to come and carried American students to flock to Paris to study under the great French masters."

very soon after the original debates took place. The editors of this journal for the most part had been students of Louis and were anxious to place before American medicine insight into these current proceedings and other developments in French medicine.

M. Francois Double was a practitioner of the old school, favoring the authority of the ancients and supporting the physician's ability to modify therapy based on the individual characteristics of his patient rather than an *arithmetical* mean obtained from the juggling of numbers.

At the time there was considerable controversy over whether mathematical treatment of clinical information was appropriate."[11]

Let M. Double speak for the large group of skeptics with a quotations from his arguments in this debate:

"The science of statistics is in these days one of the most fashionable; and in the ardor of their zeal its disciples have applied it indiscriminately to medicine.... If (it) ever be effected, medicine would cease to be either a science, an art or even a profession: <u>it would become as mechanical as the employment of the shoemaker.</u>"

M. Double continues with one of his major points, "<u>Each of our problems embraces but one individual and besides, diseases always have their prevailing</u>

[11] Article 46, The inapplicability of statistics to the practice of medicine, *Am J of the Med Sci*, XXI ,1837, p.,247-250

character, varying progressively according to an infinite variety of causes."

And how would Pierre Louis answer this blistering attack of M. Double on the duty of the practitioner to respect the individual variation in patients and the weight of past medical practice, tempered with his own knowledge and experience?

Pierre Louis begins his argument with a straight forward declaration , "A therapeutic agent cannot be employed with any discrimination or probability of success in a given case, unless its general efficacy in analogous cases has been previously ascertained:

"therefore I conceive that without the aid of statistics[12] nothing like real medical science is possible." In conclusion, Louis states, "the numerical analysis which is of no use without numerous and well observed facts, must in turn have a great influence in rendering perfect the observation of fact."

Such debates revolved around whether clinical medicine was an art dealing with the individual patient as suggested by Double or required an empirical approach with groups of patients, as suggested by Louis. If William Osler had been at these debates is it possible he would have sided more with Double in the importance of the individual patient against numerical results from groups of patients?

---

[12] As originally defined as a "science of facts concerned solely with collecting numerical data." Rosen, George, Problems in the Application of Statistical Analysis to Question of Health: 1700-1880, Bulletin of the History of Medicine 29, 1953, p. 36.

Louis' study on bleeding in pneumonia did not have a comparison group of non-treatment patients that would have made his conclusions more compelling, but considering the weight of authority that bleeding had in inflammatory conditions at that time it probably would have been impossible to have had such a controlled group. Ironically von Helmont's text of 1649 which William Osler conjured up with reference to *"a bloody Molock presides in the chairs of medicine,"* had suggested such a prospective clinical trial.[13] Von Helmont was opposed to bleeding himself primarily on basis of religious argument that the blood was the site of the soul.[14] Pierre Louis as well described a hypothetical study involving two comparable groups of patients, as in an epidemic, arbitrarily treating one group with one form of therapy and the other with a different mode and

---

[13] Niebyl, Peter H., Galen, Van Helmont, and Blood Letting , p. 19 in Science and Society in the Renaissance, Essays to honor Walter Pagel, Edited by Allen G. Debus, vol. 2 Science History publications, N.Y. 1972 Quoting Van Helmont in the Ortus medicinae of 1648, *"Let us take out of the hospitals, out of the camps, or from elsewhere, 100 or 500 poor people, that have fevers, pleurisies, etc. Let us divide them into halfes, let us cast lots, that one halfe of them may fall to my share, and the other to yours: I will coure them without blood-letting and sensible evacuation; but do you do as ye know...we shall se how many funeral both us shall have"* No such placebo controlled study was performed by Van Helmont.

[14] Bible, Deuteronomy 12:23,"For the blood is life" and Leviticus 17:11, " For the life of the flesh is in the blood..."

comparing the results.[15] Neither of these suggested studies were ever carried out however. A controlled therapeutic trial was carried out on May 1747 by the Scotchman James Lind aboard the *Salisbury* to evaluate treatment of scurvy with unequivocal results using two oranges and one lemon.[16]

Let us consider some background of the medical career of Pierre Louis and how it was a factor leading to his questioning of the value of blood letting in pneumonia.

Pierre Charles Alexandre Louis (1787 – 1872)
Background

The Paris school of medicine prepared Louis for his studies on treatment of pneumonia as well as his work on tuberculosis, yellow fever and typhoid fever. Louis came rather late to his role as a

---

[15] Louis, P.C.A., Researches on the Effects of Bloodletting in some Inflammatory Diseases, translated by C. G. Putnam (Boston, Hillaird, Gray and Co. 1836, pp.59-60. "In any epidemic, for instance, let us suppose 500 of the sick, taken indiscriminately, to be treated in a different mode: if the mortality is greater among the first than among the second, must we not conclude that the treatment was less appropriate or less efficacious in the first class, than in the second.?"

[16] Lind's Treatise on the Scurvy , 1753. p. 145-147. Lind reports taking " twelve patients in the scurvy...their cases were as similar as I could have them." Diet was all the same. There were only two subjects in each of six groups, including one with a quart of cider daily, two others given elixir of vitriol, two give vinegar, and two a course of sea-water, another with nutmeg with a electuary (laxative) of garlic and mustard seed and the only group that showed improvement, two oranges and one lemon. Of these groups the only one to show improvement was "one those who had taken them [orange and lemon} being at the end of six days [was] fit for duty. The other deemed pretty well, was appointed nurse to the rest of the sick."

clinical scientist, having spent several years in Russia as a clinician following graduation from medical school. He became troubled by the meager medical knowledge available to manage children with diphtheria and returned to France determined to spend the next seven years just observing and evaluating the course and treatment of a variety of illnesses.

He was helped in this endeavor by his contemporaries Andral and Chomel who provided him space in the hospitals to evaluate the clinical course and treatment of a number of conditions.

Louis' Studies with Bloodletting in Pneumonia

Louis originally published his observation on the treatment of pneumonia as *Memoires et Observations*[17] in 1828 where 78 patients at the hospital *la Pitie* were studied. This is the opening page of the *Memoires* with a table of results where are tabulated 50 of the patients that survived, 28 were fatal and discussed later. More legible is the table from the expanded publication of 1835, *Researches on the Effect of Bleeding in Some Inflammatory Diseases*, translated into English in the following year by C.G. Putnam with additional studies by James Jackson.[18] The figures on the horizontal line above the columns indicate the day bleeding began after onset. The figures to the left in

---

[17] Louis, PCA. *Recherche sur les effets de la saignee dans plurieurs maladies inflammatories, Archives Generales de Medecine* 1928, 18, p. 321-336

[18] Louis, PCA, Researches on the effects of bloodletting in some inflammatory disease. (Putnam, CG, transl) Boston: Hilliad, Gray and Company, 1836.

each column mark the duration of the disease, as defined by Louis, those to the right the number of bleedings, and those on the horizontal line below show on the left the mean duration of the disease and to the right the average number of bleedings.

Louis grouped together those bleed during the first two days of illness as representing *early bloodletting* (6 patients) and the remaining 44 patients bleed later in their course, third through the ninth day, *late bloodletting*. The length of the illness in these very few patients (6) who were bled early averaged eleven days, much shorter than the mean of 20.3 day for those bleed later.

This reduced length of illness may have been a factor leading to William Olser's recommendation for bleeding early in pneumonia. Remember Osler dictum, "To be of service bleeding should be done early."

However Louis is very quick to comment on this finding, recognizing that the sample size was too small and if more cases had been examined these differences "would have been considerably less."

In addition he considered that those admitted later in the course of the illness had "committed errors of regimen, strong drink and brandy, resulting in increase in the length of the disease", making the average length of illness of those bleed late, 20.3 days, falsely long.

Louis then resorts to an alternative interpretation of the data, "so that we should get nearer the truth "—by taking the mean duration of the disease in cases bled during the four first days: and on the other (hand) in those who were not bled until the fifth to the ninth inclusive. Then the mean duration of pneumonitis would be seventeen days among the first group, bleed early and twenty days among the second group bleed later." Louis has changed the definition of early from the first two days to the first four days, because the number of subjects from days one and two were small. The difference between bleeding early and late with this alternative definition of early bleeding leads to a less striking difference, average duration by new definition, 17 days as compared to later, 20 days for those bleed later.

Louis' efforts to Insure Comparability of the Group of Patients

Louis was very careful to indicate that the groups were comparable, that the "violence of the disease" and character of treatment was "equally energetic and directed by the same physician." He also was careful to note that the severity of the disease was comparable in the two groups, considering the physical findings in the chest such as "crepitation, resonance of voice, egophony, dullness on percussion as well as acceleration of pulse, 'heats' and sweats." He judged the onset of disease as the onset of fever and appearance of "pain on one side of the chest and rusty sputum; and I have regarded as the time of convalescence the period at which the sick began to take some light nourishment , three days at least after the febrile action had ceased.

Louis discusses the progression of each of these particular symptoms and signs and found little alteration following bleeding. He concludes, "that the utility of bleeding has been very limited in the cases thus far analyzed."

Fatal Cases

Louis next discusses the 28 fatal cases. Remember William Osler dictum "Pneumonia is one of the diseases in which a timely venesection may save lives" which does not seem to be well supported by the following results.

Of the patients bleed in the first four day, the alternative definition of early the early group, 18 died out of a total of 41 or 3/7 (43 %), while whose bleed later, after the 4th day, nine died of the 36 or only one quarter (25%).

Louis considered that this higher mortality in the early treated group was related to age of patients, the earlier treated group had a mean age was 41 and that of the later group 38.

Louis concludes, "Thus the study of the general and local symptoms, the mortality and variations in the mean duration of the pneumonitis, according to the period at which bloodletting was instituted; all establish narrow limits to the utility of this mode of treatment."

And then as a final point, Louis considers sarcastically the questions, "Should we obtain more important (more favorable) results if, as is practiced in England, the first bleeding were carried to syncope?"[19] Marshall Hall in England to whom Louis had dedicated his Researches, had recommended near syncope as a guide to dosing bleeding in various conditions.

Use of Statistics in Louis' Data

Louis' paper evaluated a procedure considered sacred from the time of Hippocrates, sitting abreast a most enthusiastic period for massive bleeding and leeching as proposed by Broussaais at that time for almost every medical condition. Considering the climate of the times he was remarkable for his audacity to question bleeding in an inflammatory disease.

Louis, however recognized that the relative small number of patients treated limited the significance of his conclusions. In addition there were no control groups, only averages and means.

This was not because the French didn't have the basic background in such mathematical studies.

French mathematicians such as Laplace, Fournier, and Poisson had applied theory of probability to gaming, astronomical, mortality and population studies.

---

[19] See Marshall Hall, Researches Principally related to the Morbid and Circulatory Effects of Loss of Blood, 1830 where a trial of bleeding to "near syncope" is recommended because of the varying responses to bleeding depending on the underlying diagnosis. Marshall was a close friend of Louis, with whom he communicated and visited frequently and to whom he dedicated his *Researches on the Effect of Bleeding in Inflammatory Disorders*

As a physician dedicated to careful collection and organization of clinical data Louis can perhaps be excused for not applying the then known mathematical theory to medical data where it had never been applied before.

Jules Gavarret a physician with mathematical training had applied probability calculations to Louis' mortality data to his studies in typhoid fever and indicated a lack of validity because of the limited number of observations.[20]

As pointed out by Alvan R. Feinstein, " As a pioneer in clinical statistics, Louis helped end the popularity of blood-letting by counting and comparing the results of patients treated in various ways. His general statistical techniques had many defects.... only with the advent of antibiotics to treat infectious disease, medical statistics finally reached the era of the therapeutic clinical trial." [21] This was however over 100 years after Louis' original observations.

Possible Explanations for Osler's Continued Recommendations for Bleeding in Pneumonia

The task remains to reconcile Osler's acknowledgement and praise of Pierre Louis' *methode numerique* with faint damming of his recommendations for bleeding in pneumonia. Let us consider several possible explanations for

---

[20] Gaverret, Jules, Principes generaux de satistique medicale, 1840, as discussed in chapter Louis' Numerical Method p.31, Quantification and the Quest for Medical Certainty, Matthews, J. Rosser, Princeton University Press, 1995 p. 30-33.

[21] Feinstein, Alvan R., Clinical Judgment, p.220, 222, 1967.

Osler's justification for early bleeding in pneumonia.

He could have invoked Gavarret's 1840 criticism of the validity of Louis' data where statistical theory is applied, but there is no indication that Olser was acquainted with this criticism.

Or perhaps Osler's focus on the individual patient, physician's experience and judgment as emphasized by Double in the debates may have tempered his acceptance of numerical data obtained from groups of patients?

Alternately Osler might have seen in pneumonia a component of heart failure indicating bleeding. He lists in his text book other conditions not only heart failure but cerebral hemorrhage and hypertension, or increased "arterial tension" as he called it , where bleeding is recommended.[22] Until

---

[22] From the first edition of the Principles and Practice of Medicine, 1992, Osler recommended bleeding in Arteriosclerosis, p.670 with symptoms of dyspnea and signs of cardiac insufficiency, Cerebral hemorrhage, to reduce arterial tension , Emphysema, p. 549, in a state of urgent dyspnea with engorgement of neck veins", Heart disease, p. 624, with valvular heart disease, aortic insufficiency with signs of venous engorgement. Also in sun stroke p. 1019, "...in which symptoms are those of intense asphyxia and in which death may take place in a few minutes, free bleeding should be practiced, a procedure which saved Weir Mitchell when a young man. And condemning bleeding in Yellow fever, "Careful nursing and a symptomatic plan of treatment probably gives the best results. Bleeding has long since been abandoned" Then he critically cites the "heroic procedure of Rush where 144 oz of blood at 12 bleedings in six days taken from a newly arrived Englishman, having the courage and conviction of a Sangrado, a take off on *saingree*. ? bleeding (a charlatan physician in Alain Rene Lesage novel of 1747, *Le Historie de Gil Blas de Santellane who believed in vigorous bleeding and ingestion of large quantities of warm water))*

potent diuretics were developed bleeding was an accepted treatment of severe heart failure. A recent unpublished paper by our chairman, Dr. Charles S. Bryan et al, *Bloodletting for Pneumonia: Closure to a Controversy*, reviewed the data that supports the findings that perhaps one quarter of patients with pneumonia may have evidence of heart failure.

Or did William Osler's emphasis on Louis' contribution and influence on training a group of physicians who created an American school of clinical medicine trump the importance of the results of the *methode numerique* in initiating the demise of bleeding in pneumonia ?[23]

Osler and subsequent editors continued to recommend bleeding in pneumonia throughout subsequent editions of the *Principles and Practice of Medicine* through 1944.

Major Greenwood has considered that, "Louis indeed seemed more honoured in America than France and Osler honoured him not so much as the inventor of the numerical method as the teacher of the Americans such as James Jackson, , Bowditch, Oliver Wendell Homes and William Gerhard."[24] This appraisal is somewhat confirmed by Arnold C. Klebs who accompanied Osler to Louis' mausoleum at the Montparnasse Cemetery in 1905

---

[23] Richard H. Shryock came to a similar conclusion in his book, *The Development of Modern Medicine*, 1936 in a footnote on p. 160, "Osler, despite the tribute in his essay on Louis' Influence on American Medicine saw him only as a representative of the French clinical school."

[24] Greenwood, Major, The Medical Dictator, in the chapter, Louis and the Numerical Method, p.123, 1936.

recalling Osler's actual remarks , "Louis has a far higher claim on our affection and gratitude, as through his students he may have be said to have created the American school of clinical medicine." [25] Such was Olser's assessment of Louis and as for his results in his *Researches on the Effect of Bloodletting in Pneumonia*, they are not mentioned at the tomb that day.

At the time of the American's visit to Louis' tomb, Pierre Louis' reputation had fallen to such a low points that according to Cushing in his biography of Osler,[26] "no one, not even the French physicians who were consulted, had any idea where Louis was buried." Cushing added to Osler's remarks as remembered by Klebs at the tomb, noting "the sad death of his son at the age of eighteen from tuberculosis, of his [Louis'] own death from the same disease at the age of eighty –five; of his special claims to remembrance - not so much his attempt to introduce mathematical accuracy into the study of disease, [but] his higher claim to have created the American school of clinical medicine through his pupils." Erwin Ackerknecht summarized Louis' bitter sweet later life, "He was condemned to live to a very advanced age, and to be the sad survivor of his young son, his dearest pupils such as Jackson, his closest friends like Chomel and Marshall Hall, and of his own importance. [27]

---

[25] Klebs, A.C. Osler at the Tomb of Louis, JAMA, Vol. 16, 1906, p.1916-1917. Osler's actual words as quoted by Klebs

[26] Cushing, Harvey, The Life of Sir William Olser, p 706-707, 1940.

[27] Ackerknecht, Erwin H., Medicine at the Paris Hospital 1794-1848 p.103, 1967.

Summary

Background on Pierre Louis' studies on bleeding in pneumonia showing "narrow limits to the utility of this mode of treatment."

Debates at the Royal Academy of Medicine on the applicability of statistics to medicine

Evaluation of Louis's results in treating 78 patients with pneumonia with bloodletting

Lack of statistical methods applied by Louis to his studies in spit of French mathematician's studies in gaming, astronomy and mortality tables.

Discussion of reasons for William Osler's continued recommendations for bleeding in pneumonia in spite of his labeling Louis' method *iconoclastic,* writing an essay on his contributions to American medicine and visiting his grave in 1905.

Systeme de Broussais   Broussais intructs a nurse to extract even more blood from a pallid patient with leeches on his chest and blood dripping from all over his body.

　　　　Patient: " But I have no more than a drop of blood in my veins."
　　　　Broussais: " Never mind, 50 more leeches."

Historical AfterNote

Let us consider a brief historical sketch of what is called bloodletting, later in history enacted by the use of leaches. Blood letting had been employed by medicine since antiquity. It is even debated as therapeutic in the Talmud (Yoma 84a). The Talmud expresses the merit of a bloodletter named Abba (Taanith 21b) named Abba who had separate rooms for men and women but also insisted that women wear a special garment he had so that only the site of bloodletting was exposed. The mention of blood letting is also found in the secular texts as well (oelius Auelianus, Acut. 3 chapter 4:34, p. 193). The Talmud further notes that Nebuchadnezzar chose for himself young people without blemish which the Talmud explains "there was not even a lancet puncture on their bodies" (Sanhr. 93b). Maimonides 1135-1204 recognized that routine phlebotomy is not advised and certainly after the age of fifty it is prohibited (Misheh Torah Hilchot Deot 4:18). The Talmud uses the terms lancet as Kusulha or perhaps scariffum. Rashi uses the old French phrase of pointure de flieme or a prick of the lancet. Another method blood letting was the use of cupping glasses. Known by the Talmud as keren or coru (horn). Whereas the physician in Judaism is a chakham, the bloodletter in the Talmud as his name of umman or ummana connotes an artisan sometimes called gara (Kiddushin 82a; Kelim12:4; Derech eretz Zutta 10:2), wich is the meaning of the Latin expression minutor. Latin gara is minuens sanguinem. In Syriac minuens barbam, the cutter or barber. The functions of the barber were served by the sappur. The umman refers to the Greek aimon which means shedder of blood (i.e. murderer) is not established as a clear etymology. The Mishnah commentator Rabbi Ovadia Bartenura mentions the interpretation of blacksmith. While the doctor or rophe from the root to heal in Hebrew could do surgical acts the blood letter sometimes as a different position. However a rophe who also did blood letting may be indicated by the phrase rophe umman.

Chapter Three

Colour Indicators, Robert Boyle's *"Experimental History of Colours,"* and Lignum nephriticum

Introduction

Pierre Rayer in the first volume of his *Traite des Maladies des Reins* in the Prolegemenon under ***Alterations de l'urine – degre'd'acidite*** (alterations of the urine – degree of acidity) states, *"To determine the degree of acidity of the urine --- you mix a certain measure of urine with some **infusion of tournesol** "*, *noting the amount of ammonia required to turn the red colour of the tournesol to blue, indicating the presence of acid, thus determining the degree of acidity of the urine."*[1] This procedure sounds like the modern version of determining tritable acidity, but what is this **tournsesol** in the place of a pH meter we might currently use for this determination? Tournesol as French speaking person knows is the name for sun flower; ie., turning toward the sun. Actually what was used in the France in the 18th and 19th century was not sunflower but a related

---

[1] Rayer, Pierre F. O. , Traite des Maladies des Reins, Tome I, p. 87.

plant that is also a heliotrope, *Crozophora tinctoria,* that grows on sunny, well drained Mediterranean slopes.[2] It was this three-lobed fruit, not the leaves, that were used from the thirteenth century on as the mainstay of medieval manuscript illumination as well as dying fabrics.[3]

The dyers of that time in order to obtain blue coloring used this plant placed at the bottom of a dye vat, soaking the clothes to be dyed in a closed, damp cellar in an alkaline atmosphere produced by pans of urine that produced ammonia turning the tournesol alkaline, thereby producing varying degrees of blue.[4] This was a procedure of the dyer's art, although they did not realize that they were taking advantage of the plant's ability to change from red to blue with pH change from acid to alkaline. Robert Boyle in the seventeenth century however was instrumental in characterizing and systematizing these color changes of the dyers art. This allowed Rayer in the early nineteenth century to determine titratability acidity, using color changes described six centuries earlier with the dyer's art of the thirteenth century with a similar plant, tournesol. We still today use Litmus, which is a lichen, a symbiotic combination of an algae and fungi, to represent a pH color indicator in a similar way.

---

[2] Eamon, William, New Light on Robert Boyle and the Discovery of Colour Indicators, Abbix, Vol.27, November 1980,. Part 3, References 10, p. 208

[3] Thompson, Daniel V., The Materials and Techniques of Medieval Painting 1958, Dover Publications, pp 141-145.

[4] Ibid. p. 205.

Colour Indicators

Aristotle indicated that taste and appearance were the best determiner of the quality of mineral springs. Pliny was the first to advocate oak gall, outgrowths on trees caused by a combination of natural growth products of the tree and parasites such as fungi, insects and bacteria, to determine the purity of alum.[5] Pleny indicates that alum that is adulterated will be stained by oak gall. He does not state that it will be turned black but this is suggested. Oak galls contain tannic and gallic acids and yield clear fluid, which if combined with an iron salt, produces a purplish-black compound which in the middle ages was used as an ink in many early manuscripts.[6] Paracelsus described the oak-galls test in one of his earliest works according

---

[5] Pliny, Natural History, Book XXXV, 1 184-185, Huius quoque duae species, liquidum spissumque. Liquidi probation ut sit limpidum lacteumque,sine offensi fricandi, cum quodam igniculo coloris. Hoc phorimon vocant. An sit adulteratulm , deprehenditur suco Punici mali; sincerum enim mixture ea non nigreseit. Alterum genus est pallidi et scabri et quod inficiatur et galla, (The test of the fluid kind is that it should be of a limpid, milky consistency, free from grit when rubbed between the fingers, and giving a slight glow of colour; this kind is called in Greek "phorimon" in the sense of abundant. Its alteration can be detected by means of the juice of a pomegranate, as this mixed with it does not turn it black if it is pure. *The other kind (of alum) which may be stained with oak-gall also , and consequently this is called paraphoron,-perverted or adulterated alum.)*

[6] Thompson , Daniel, V, *"The Materials and Techniques of Medieval Painting,* Dover Publication, Inc. NY, NY. ,1956, p. 81. Bach used such ink –iron-gall ink in many of his manuscripts including the Cello suites and being highly acidic has lead to severe damage, "note heads falling away , leaving holes in the paper and a manuscript that resembles Swiss cheese." Siblin, Eric, *"The Cello Suites,* Atlantic Monthly Press NY, 2009, p. 269.

to Allen Debus and characterized the craft of the medieval dyers:[7]

"Medieval dyers and painters knew empirically that plants could be made to yield a wide range of colours dependent on the season of the year in which they were collected and the mordants that were used with them...The craftsmen also knew that certain colour changes could be induced chemically, for very few of the vegetable extracts in medieval technology were used in their natural state...All the plant dyes and pigments were made by combining the natural juices of plants and flowers with some acid or basic material to develop their colour. With such initial preparation, and by treating the textiles with different mordants, a variety of shades and sometimes even different colours could be obtained from a single dyestuff."[8]

The turnsol plant (Crozophora tinctoria) a versatile agent that could be manipulated to give a variety of colors depending on whether acid such as vinegar or alkali, often in the form of stale urine that yielded an alkaline agent, was often used as noted above. Robert Boyle was familiar with the dyers of his day who empirically produced a wide variety of colours with various plant sources and this was his starting point in developing a chemical basis for these reactions. He studied violets and a variety of other plants as well as the wood from the new world, Lignum nephriticum.

---

[7] Debus, Allen G. , Solution Analyes Prior to Robert Boyle, Chymia 8, 1962, p. 45.

[8] Eamon, William. New Light on Robert Boyle and the Discovery of Colour Indicators, Ambix, Fol 27. Part3, November 1980, p.204 and 205.

Robert Boyle

Robert Boyle of Boyle's gas law which we learned in high school (volume and pressure of a gas are inversely related) and one of the founders of the Royal Society, was also intrigued by color changes in a variety of plants and especially in this wood from Mexico called *Lignum Nephriticium*. The wood had been admired and considered a remedy for a variety of kidney conditions for centuries before the Spanish naturalists in the mid sixteenth century traveling to *Neuva Espana (New Spain or Mexico)* described. a beautiful blue color obtained when clear pure liquid was allowed to mix with slices of the white slices of this tree, called by Aztez Indians, *Coatli.*

SPANISH NATURALIST : MONARDES AND JOHN FRAMPTON'S TRANSLATION

Who were these Spanish naturalist and explorers who brought back news about the New World plants such as Tobacco, Peper (pepper), Guaiacan, Sinamon (cinnamon), Coca, Sassafras and Sarsaparilla as well as Ginger? The first person to write about these agents was Dr. Nicolas Monardes, a physician, in his book *Dos Libros* or in Latin *De Libris Simplicissimis ex India Allatis , 1565-69 (The Most Basic Book Gathered from India).* Unlike other explorers to be described, Monardes never left his home of Seville in southern Spain.[9] But is was this location that allowed him to examine the many specimens brought back from *Neuva Espana,* since it

---

[9] Boxer, C.R., Two Pioneers of Tropical Medicine: Garcia D'Orta and Nicolas Monardes, Wellcome Historical Medical Library, London, N. W. 1, 1963, Lecture Series No. 1.

was the major seaport where such material was delivered to Spain. He planted the material coming to this port in his garden and made observations. Tobacco was planted primarily for its large leaves enhancing the appearance of the garden as well as its medicinal use in healing wounds.[10] His book was immensely popular and within several years of its publication was translated into Latin, French and into English by John Frampton, a West County merchant formerly living in Spain who had been imprisoned and tortured by the Inquisition before making his escape from Cadiz in 1567. The English title of his book was labeled *Joyfvll Nevves Out of the Newe Founde Worlde,* published in 1577. While reading this fascinating book, and while easier that the Spanish, it was almost just as difficult because of the Chaucer- like spelling of many of the words. Indeed it is Monardes in the Latin edition that is quoted by Boyle who begins his discussion of *Lignum Nephriticum*[11] after this introduction:

"The ancientest Account I have met with of this Simple ("a medicine composed or concocted of only one constituent")[12], *is given us by the Experience'd Monardes in these Words."* Boyle then begins   in

---

[10] Monardes, Nicolas, Dos Libros 1565, as translated into English by John Frampton, *"Of the Tabaco, and of his Greate Vertues,* p.75. *"Within this few yeres there hath beene brought to Spaine of it, more to adornate Gardeines with the fairenes thereof, and to geve a pleasaunt sight, rather, then that whiche it hath, now we doe use of it more for his vertues, then for his fairenes."*

[11] Boyle, Robert, The Beginning of an Experimental History of Colours,, 1664, p. 76, in the Echo Library, edition of 2007.

[12] Definition from the Oxford English Dictionary. 1646 Sir T. Brown, "From the knowledge of Simples she has a Receipt to make white hair black."

Latin which I will render into the English of John Frampton translation: *"Of the Woodde for the Evilles of the Raines, and of the Urine,* describing the details of the production of this blue colour from clear water placed in contact with white wood:

"Also thei doe bryng from the new Spaine, a certaine woodde that is like unto the woodd of a Peare tree, grosse and without knottes: the whiche thei have used thereof many yeres in that partes, for the paines of the Raines, and of the Stone and for the infirmities of the Urine... Thei doe take the woode, and doe make it in small peeces verie thinne, and small as it is possible, and thei putte theim into cleare water of the Fountaine, whiche is verie good and cleare, and thei leave it so until the water bee sokened into it: and in puttyng the wooded into the Water, within halfe an hower the water doeth beginne to chaunge it self into a blewe couller verie cleare and the longer that it lieth in the water, so muche the Blewer it tourneth, although that the woode bee of a white couller."[13]

Boyle perhaps because he wasn't a physician and more interested in the details of the production of that *"blewe couller verie cleare,"* neglects to quote Monardes' further interesting additional clinical information which is supplied in John Frampton's translation, *Of the Wodde for the Evilles of the Raines, and of the Urine* :

"the firste tyme that I sawe it used (maie bee aboute XXXV yeres paste) there was a Pilot that was sicke of the Urine and of the Raines, and after that he had used

---

[13] Boyle, Robert, the Beginning of an Experimental History of Colours 1664, Echo Library edition 2007. p. 76.

it, he was whole and very well. And sithence that tyme I have seen that many have brought it from the newe Spain, and thei doe use it for these remedies.

Frampton continues his translation of Menardes of the alleged benefits of this blue liquid which is not quoted by Boyle:

"For them that doeth not pisse liberally, and for the paines of the Raines, and of the stone, and for theim that doeth pisse with paine, and for them that dooeth pise little. And now the thing hath extended for opilations, for that the water thereof doeth cure and heale them and also of the Lunges and the Liver, and this hath been founde within these few yeres thei doe finde in it notable profite. The water is made in this forme.

The Latin translation of Monardes which was used by Bolye was by Charles de L'Ecluse (Feb 18.1525 – April 4 1609) linguist, physician and botanist from Holland who gave the Mexican tree the Latin name, Lignum nephriticum whereas the Mexican name was Coatli.

Monardes' book that yields an equally interesting account concerning the Guaican tree: "Of The Guaiacan, and of the Holie Woodde" as translated by Frampton[14]: This was used for the pox or syphilis which Monardes recognized as a disease the Spanish acquired from the Indians. This alleged remedy was described by Benvenuto Cellini, sixteenth century Italian goldsmith and sculpturer

---

[14] Monardes, N. as translated by Frampton, *Joyfull Newes Out of the Newfound World – Of the Guaiacan, and of the Holie Woodde. P. 28--33.*

in his autobiography.[15] We used the guiac to test for fecal blood for many years.

FRANCISCO HERNADEZ EXPLORER OF NUEVA ESPANA

A contemporary of Monardes, who remember never came to Mexico, was Francisco Hernandez, the Mexican explorer who spent seven years in Nueva Espana.[16] He was a physician at the Escorial and the court of Philipp 11 of Spain. In 1570 he was commissioned by the king to explore Nueva Espana and report on the flora and fauna of the country. He brought back with him a tremendous amount of notes, twenty four volumes, illustrations and information which he placed in the library of the Escorial but it was never published apparently because of funds for that

---

[15] The Life of Benvenuto Cellini, an autobiography translated by John Addington Symonds, chapter 59, p.108, 1953. "It was true indeed that I had got the sickness, but I believed I caught it from the fine young servant girl whom I was keeping when my house was robbed. The French disease (syphilis), for it was that, remained in me more than four months dormant before it showed itself, and then it broke out over my whole body at on instant. It was not like what one commonly observes, but covered my flesh with certain blisters, of the size of sixpences, and rose-colored. The doctors would not call it the French disease, albeit I told them why I thought it was that. I went on treating myself according to their methods, but derived no benefit. At last-I resolved on taking the wood (Guaiacum) against the advice of the first physicians in Rome, and I took it with the most scrupulous discipline and rules of abstinence that could be thought of, and after a few days, I perceived in me a great amendment. The result was that at the end of fifty days I was cured and as sound as a fish in the water."

[16] Stapf, Otto, Lignum nephriticum, Bulletin of the Miscellaneous Information (Royal Gardens, Kew)), Vol 1909. No.1 7 (1909). Pp. 293-305.

purpose where not available and Hernandez died nine years later a broken man. King Philipp 11 appointed his next physician, Nardo Antonio Recchi of Naples to prepare an abstract of Hernandes' findings, but again this was never published, but found its ways to Rome where it was eventually partially published in 1651. In 1671 there was a fire in the Escorial and Hernandez original manuscript was completely destroyed. Other versions of Hernandez original work prepared by Gomez Ortega have been found and he comments on the shrub or tree called Coatl, chips of the trunk yield *"an azure blue colour, and if drunk it refreshes and relieves the kidneys and the bladder, alleviates the acidity of the urine, extinguishes fever, heals colic pains, and is does all this with great force and efficiency."*[17]

Other description of the wood whose infusion gave a blue color and was helpful in kidney conditions have been described by others from fragments of Hernandes' original report found in various places. The relationship of the wood, blue color and kidney disease may have originated as indicated by Otto Stapf from the report of a Spanish bishop that the "kidney shape of the seeds of this plant indicated that it was to be used in diseases of the kidney as well as the fact about the seeds was a "white poppy substance" that resembled the fat about the kidneys." [18]

ROBERT BOYLE'S *THE BEGINNING OF AN EXPERIMENT HISTORY OF COLOURS, 1664*

---

[17] Ibid, p. 297.

[18] Ibid. p. 300.

Robert Boyle in his book, *The Beginning of An Experimental History of Colours, 1664,* describes in his introduction to Lignum nephriticum:

"We have sometimes found in the Shops of our Druggists, a certain Wood which is there called Lignum Nepriiticum, because the Inhabitants of the Country where it grows, are wont to use the Infusion of it made in fair Water against the Stone of the Kidneys, and indeed an Eminent Physician of our Acquaintance who has very Particularly enquir'd into that Disease, assures me, that he has found such an Infusion one of the most effectual Remedyes, which he has ever tried against that Formidable. Disease."[19]

Boyle gives us no further medical insight into the usefulness of this blue liquid, but as the father of modern chemistry concentrated his interest in color changes in various plants, syrup of violets, Tounsol as well as Lignum nephriticum. He utilized the knowledge of color changes by dyers and painters who empirically knew that under different conditions plants would change their color with the addition of acids or alkali. He had some vinegar which he knew was an acid and on adding a few drops to the caeruleous fluid found that the "deep and lovely Caeruleous colour,"[20] entirely disappeared only to be reinvigorated into that same blue color with the addition of an agent he considered an alkali. An agents that he considered as salts had no effect on the color:

---

[19] Boyle, Robert, The Beginning of An Experimental History of Colours, 1664, p, 76, Echo Library edition, 2007

[20] Ibid, p. 77.

"whereupon Pouring into a small Vial full of Impregnated Water, a very little Spirit of Vinegar, I found that according to my Expectation, the Caeruleous Colour immediately vanish'd.......Upon this I imagin'd that the Acid Salts of the Vinegar having been able to deprive the Liquor of its Caeruleous Colour, a Suphureus Salt (alkali) *being of a contrary Nature, would be able to Mortifie the Saline Particles of Vinegar, and Destroy their Effects. And accordingly having plac'd my self betwixt the Window and the vial, and into the Same Liquorr dropt a few drops of Oyle of Tartar* (an alkali) *I observ'd with pleasure, that immediately upon the Diffusion of this Liquor, the Impregnated Water was restor'd to its former Caeruleus Colour."*[21]

Boyle continues as to the practical usefulness of these observations:

"That this Experiment... may be as well Usefull as Delightfull to You,...I have hinted to You a New and Easie way of Discovering in many Liquors (for I dare not say in all) whether it be an Acid or Sulphureous Salt (an alkali) *that is predominant; and that such a Discovery is oftentimes of great Difficulty, and may frequently be of great Use, he that is not a Stranger to the various Properties and Effects of Salts, and of how great moment it is to be able to distinguish their Tribes*(this group of substances), *may readily conceive."*

Bolye then gives an example of the usefulness of this procedure using an unknown substance, Alum, the same substance evaluated by Pliny :

---

[21] Ibid,, p.78.

"I turn my back to the Light, and holding a small Vial full of the Tincture of _Lignum Nephriticum_, which look'd upon in that Position, appears Caeruleous, I drop into a little of a strong Solution of Allom(alum – astringent properties, AlK(SO4) *made in Fair Water, and finding upon the Affusion* (pouring) *and shaking of this New liquor, that the Blewness formerly conspicuous in our Tincture does presently vanish, I am thereby incited to suppose, that the Salt Predominant in Allom belongs to the Family of Sour Salts* (acids); *but if on the other side, I have a mind to examine whether or no I rightly conceive that Salt of Urine or of Harts-horn* (horns of a male red deer[22]) *is rather of a Saline Sulphureous* (alkaline) *than of an Acid Nature, I drop a little of the Saline Spirit of either into the Nephritick Tincture and finding that the Caeruleous Colour is rather thereby Deepned than Destroy'd, I collect that the Salts, which constitute these Spirits, are rather Sulphureous* (alkaline).[23]

Boyle continues, *to satisfie my self farther in this particular,* he *deprives* the *Blewness* of Lignum nephriticum with vinegar and on *drooping and shaking into the same Vial a small proportion of spirit of* Hartshorn (ammonia) *or* Urine, *the Tincture immediately recovers its Caeruleous Colour, I am thereby confirm'd my former Opinion of the Suphureous* (alkaline) *Nature of these Salts.*

---

[22] Spirits of hartshorn is an aqueous solution of ammonia made from the hooves and horns of the red deer. Hartshorn salt (ammonium carbonate) was used as a leavening agent in the baking of cookies in the 17th and 18th century as a forerunner of baking powder. Davidson, Alan (1999) Oxford Companion to Food, Oxford: Oxford University Press, p. 372.

[23] Bolye, Robert, The Beginning of an Experimental History of Colours, 1664, p. 81, Echo Library edition.

With these studies Boyle gives us the very first definition of an acid: ie., a substance that will regularly *deprive* the blue color of *Lignum Nephriticum* and of an alkali a substance that will regularly *restore* the blue color. Until that time the acid –alkali theory, supported by Helmont and others, held that the reaction between the two would always produce effervescence, as when an acid is added to an alkali such as potassium carbonate, when carbon dioxide was produced, producing effervescence.[24] However Boyle maintained that the reactions between some acids and alkali do not always produce effervescence and the ability of an acid to regularly deplete the blue colour of *Lignum nephriticum* as well as changing the blue colour of syrup of violets to red was a more appropriate criteria. While there are many more modern definitions of an acid or a alkali, this was the first and a Professor Chemistry of my acquaintance recalls the primacy of Boyles definition.

In addition Boyle was the first to cut strips of paper, impregnated with the blue liquid of *Lignum Nephriticum* and other agents such as Syrrup of Violets to determine the color change of an unknown substance, much as we would do with litmus paper today. *"Take good Syrrup of Violets, Impraegnated with the Tincture of the flowers, drop a little of it upon a White Paper (for by that means the Change of Colour will be more conspicuous and the Experiment may be practis'd in smaller Quantities) and on this Liquor let fall two or three drops of Vinegar, or almost any other eminently Acid Liquor and upon the*

---

[24] Boas, Marie, Robert Bolyle and Seventeeth-century Chemistry, 1959, p. 58.

mixture of these you shall find the Syrrup immediately turns Red..."[25]. Boyle continues this experiment with Syrrup of Violets indicating, *that " if instead of vinegar you drop upon the Syrup of Violets a little Oyl of Tartar or the like quantity of Solution of Potashes (alkaline agents) and rubb them together with your finger, you shall find the Blew Colour of the Syrrup turn'd in a moment into a perfect Green, and the like may be perform'd by divers other Liquors, a s we may have occasion elsewhere to Inform you."[26]*

Here Boyle is using a piece of white paper impregnated with *Syrrup of Violets,* much as we would use Litmus paper to first see the color change to Red on addition of an acid and back to Green on addition of an alkali.

Furthermore he considered the strength of the acid or alkali by, *"I allow my self to guess at the **Strength** of the Liquors examin'd by this Experiment, by the Quantity of them which is sufficient to Destroy or Restore the Caeruleous Colour of our Tincture." [27]*

NEWTON'S EVALUATION OF LIGNUM NEPHRITICUM

Newton also evaluated Lignum nephriticum in several places in his book on Optics, 1704, noting that the tincture has capacity of "transmitting one sort of Light most copiously and reflecting another

---

[25] Boyle, Robert, The Beginning of an Experimental History of Colours, 1664 p. 92, Echo Library edition,.

[26] Ibid. p. 92-93.

[27] Ibid. p. 82.

sort ...according to the Position of the Eye to the Light." [28] He was more interested in the physical qualities of the color then in its possible application to chemistry and defining acid and bases. Bolye also paid considerable attention to the quality of the color in his studies depending on the position of the observer and the source of light.

GEORGE G. STOKES AND FLUORESENCE

Since the work of George Gabriel Stokes (1820-1903) professor of mathematics at Cambridge, blue color exhibited by Lignum nephriticum has been designated as a phenomenon of fluorescence in 1853, that is as an emission of light during the irradiation of a substance by any type of radiation which ceases when the exciting radiation is cut off. "Florescence occurs when a substance absorbs light in one wavelength region and at the same time emits light in a different region of the spectrum, normally of longer wave length. The characteristic shift to longer wavelength from absorbed light to emitted light is known as the Stokes shift." [29] The description of the blue color from Lignum nephriticum by Monardes and studied so elegantly by Boyle from the standpoint of changes in color with acids and bases represented the first report of

---

[28] Newton, Isaac, *Opticksor, a Treatise of the Reflection, Refractions, Inflections and Colours of Light, 1740 4th edition, p184.* "there are some Liquors, as the Tincture of Lignum Nephriticum, and some sorts of Glass which transmit one sort of Light most copiously, and reflect another sot, and thereby look of several Colours, according to the Position of the Eye to the Light. Etc"

[29]Muyskens, Mark, the Fluorescence of Lignum nephriticum: A Flash Back to the Past and a Simple Demonstration of Natural Substance Fluorescence, Journal of Chemical Education, Fo. 83, No. 5, May 2005, p. 765.

fluorescence, before of course it was defined by Stokes in 1853.[30]

Evaluation of Robert Boyle's Use of Lignum nephtiticum

Marie Boas has pointed out that Boyle's tests for acids and alkali were rapidly known and accepted. "The tests were of great importance for the theory of classification, and as an argument counter to the acid-alkali theory; but their greatest importance lay in their usefulness for determining chemical composition, and for setting a precedent for the use of such tests in ordinary chemical analysis."[31]

Lawrence M. Principe has indicated that Bolye stood on the threshold between alchemy and modern chemistry.[32] While many of Boyle's writings have a flavor of the occult and on the transmutation of metals, his work on color indicators and the use he placed on *Lignum nephriticum* suggest he was clearly laying the foundations for modern chemistry. Taking the lead from his observations of the dyers of his acquaintance in their ability to modify colors in cloth with what we would call pH change he focused on the usefulness of an acid such as vinegar to regularly deprive the blue color of *Lignum nephriticum,* so defining an acid. Similarly an alkaline substance was one that would restore

---

[30] Valeur, Bernard, Molecular Fluorescence, Principles and Application, 2001, p. 5.

[31] Boas, Marie, Robert Boyle and seventeenth-Century Chemistry, Cambridge at the University Press, 1958, p.134.

[32] Principe, Lawrence M. , The Aspiring Adept, Robert Boyle and his Alchemical Quest, Princeton University Press, 1998.

the color. A salt would not affect the blue color. Not being a physician he did not evaluate it's usefulness in kidney disease as he reported of his *"Eminent Physician of our Acquaintance---who had assured me that such an Infusion was one of the most effectual Remedyes... against that formidable Disease."* These color tests would become an important foundation for establishing a scientific basis to allow modern chemistry to emerge from alchemy.

RECENT CHEMICAL EXPLANATION FOR BLUE FLUORESCENCE

The tree used by Boyle and Newton to evaluate Lignum nephriticum has become extent in the past 150 year and is no longer available.[33] More recently the Spanish chemist, A.U. Acufia and F. Amat-Guerri using a related tree have reported on the fluorescent components of Lignum nephriticum isolating coatline A that yield matlaline, a fluorophore that is pH dependent. The resonance of these organic compounds have been shown to be responsible for the blue fluorescence of Lignum nephriticum.[34]

CONTEMPARY EVALUATION OF LIGNUM NEPHRITICUM

---

[33] Stapf, Otto, Lignum nephriticum, Bulletin of Miscellaneous Information (Royal Gardens, Kew), Vol. 1909. No 7,1909, p. 293-94.

[34] Structure and Formation of the Fluorescent Compound of *Lignum nephriticum* , Acufui, Ulises, amat-Guerri, Francisco, et. al., structure and Formation of the Fluorescent Compound of Lignum nephriticum, Organic Letters, Vol. 11. No. 14, p. 3030-3023.

Finally as the efficacy of Lignum nephriticum as a therapeutic agent in diseases of the kidney has come under some questioning, inspite of being highly recommended by both Monardes as well as Boyles' "Eminent Physician" who had assured him "that he had found such an Infusion one of the most effectual Remedyes which he had ever tried in that formidable Disease." By the end of the eighteenth century Edinburgh, Scotland was the center of medical progress. The Edinburgh New Dispensatory of 1788 under Materia Medica after describing this "American wood demonstrating remarkable blue color under certain situations" and while acknowledging that it had "stood recommended in difficulties of urine, nephritic complaints and all disorders of the kidneys and urinary passages", the Dispensatory gave it its final judgement. *"Practioners however have not found these virtues warranted by experience."*[35]

Summary

The dyers and painters of the middle ages and early Renaissance used plant sources, modified empirically by various agents that changed the colours by what we would call acids or bases. Robert Boyle was familiar with these methods of the dyers of his time. The discoveries of plants and products from the New World were described most vividly by Nicolas Monardes in his book, Dos Libros of 1565-69, translated into Latin as well a into English by John Frampton under the title, *"Joyfull Newes Out of the Newfound World.* With the description of Lignum nephriticum from a tree

---

[35] The Edinburgh New Dispensatory , 1788, in section on material medica , p. 235

whose white wood would produce a beautiful caereuleous or blue color having the reputation as being helpful for all types of kidney conditions, Robert Boyle took up a study of the chemistry of color changes in a variety of plants as well as Lignum nephriticum. Boyle published his findings in *"The Beginning of an Experimental History of Colours, 1664.* His studies indicated that the blue color of Lignum nephriticum could be obliterated with not only an acid such as acetic acid from vinegar but all acids and restored by an alkali and unaffected by a salt. Bolye's defined an acid as an agent that would regularly obliterate the blue color of Lignum nephriticum which was the first definition of an acid and helped characterize acids, bases and salts. He also used strips of paper, impregnated with an infusion of Lignum nephriticum or syrup of violets and other plant agent to test substances as to whether they were acids, bases or salts. The caereuleus color of Lignum nephriticum was to be the first demonstration of fluorescence, not to be defined until 1856 by George Stokes. Therapy of Lignum nephriticum for kidney disease was recommened for centuries however the Edinburgh Dispensary or 1788 disputed such claims: *"Practitioners have not found these virtues warranted by experience."* Boyle's studies with Lignum nephriticum defined acid and bases and were an early advance in modern chemistry.

Chapter Four

Pulvis Ipecacunanhae et Opii—The Powder and the Buccaneer Thomas Dover (1660 – 1742)

The most efficient diaphoretic is Dover's Powder, 5-8 gr.
3 times a day with a warm bath.
Sir Robert Christison, On Granular Degeneration of the Kidney, 1839, p. 65.

These are the several Symptoms of an approaching Dropsy...The Thirst is more intense, Urine less in Quantity, higher coloured, coming near to the Water made in a Jaundice; shortness of Breath to that Degree, that there is no lying down in Bed; an Inability to all Motions; a total loss of Appetite. The Legs, thighs and all Parts of the Body, are full of Water; which make up the frightful   merciless Retinue that attend this great Evil. Let me but come to People as early in this Distemper, as they generally apply for Relief from other Physicians, and it shall be cured with as much Certainty as any other Gentleman may cure a Distemper he thinks himself most Master of. Thomas Dover, The Ancient Physician's Legacy to his Country, 6th

Edition 1742, p.19-20, facsimile edition of Kenneth Dewhurst 1974.

Dover's powder, introduced in 1740, has been in the Pharmacopoeia for over 200 hundred years. It is usually considered a mixture of opium and ipecac and while originally prescribed as an antidote to the gout, has usually been considered as a sweating or diaphoretic agent. Sir William Osler, known as a therapeutic conservative, mentions the use of Dover's powder in his *Principles and Practice of Medicine*[1]. In his chapter on typhoid fever, after initially promulgating his well known dictum, "The profession was long in learning that typhoid fever is not a disease to be treated mainly with drugs", Osler advocates Dover's powder, not as a diaphoretic agent but to counteract diarrhea. He also recommends its use for similar circumstances in tuberculosis, as well as in rheumatic fever to alleviate pain. Osler read a paper on Thomas Dover, *The Physician and Buccaneer* at the Johns Hopkins Historical Club in January 1895,[2] which deals with Thomas Dover's career as a sea captain and buccaneer as well as his activities as a physician.

Dover was born in Barton-on-Heath, in the Cotswold, educated at both Oxford and Cambridge, took an apprenticeship with Thomas Sydenham. He was a fellow student with Hans

---

[1] Osler William, The Principles and Practice of Medicine eight edition, 1916.

[2] Ibid, reprinted in An Alabama Student, p.19-36. While buccaneer has become equated with a pirate, the term comes from the French word, *Boucanier*, originally referring to the smoking of meat on wooden frames, *boucans*, by hunters on Santo Domingo, who later took to pirating activities.

Sloane, a less controversial figure and collector of art and other items that became the founding core of the British Museum, as well as becoming President of the Royal Society and the College of Physicians. Dover then settled in Bristol to begin his practice of medicine. At the age of forty-six he took to sea as a captain and doctor, in 1708 to raid Spanish settlements and capture Spanish ships.[3] Bristol was the second largest seaport in England and famous for its expeditions to the New World. A group of merchants, including Dover who had a financial interest in the project, outfitted two ships, the *Duke* and the *Dutchess*. The project participated in many adventures, gathered considerable loot, as well as rescuing Alexander Selkerk, a Scotchman who had been stranded on a South Sea island for three and one half years and who became the model for Defoe's Robinson Crusoe. After three years at sea, having circumnavigated the globe Dover returned to England, much wealthier for his adventures and settled in London resuming his role as a physician.

In 1732 Dover wrote a popular book on medical treatment entitled *The Ancient Physician's Legacy to his Country*,[4] having eight subsequent printings through 1771. On the title page is stated, *an Account of the several Diseases incident to Mankind; described in so plain a Manner, That any person may know the Nature of his own Disease together with the several Remedies for each distemper, faithfully set down.*

[3] Phear, D.N., Thomas Dover 1662-1742, Physician, Privateering Captain, and Inventor of Dover's powder, Journal of the History of Medicine and Allied Sciences, Inc.,Volume IX p. 139-156, 1954.

[4] From the 6th edition as published in facsimile by Dewhust, Kenneth, Thomas Dover's Life and Legacy 1974.

Designed for the use of all Private Families. The book made a great commotion among the coffee houses of London, because it was primarily a manual for patient's use to treat their own diseases or *distempers,* as Dover calls them. The braggadocio of the old Buccaneer's style and his truculent manner of dealing with colleagues who disagreed with his methods contributed to the controversy. Perhaps the most over-the-top tale is his description of an epidemic of plague on board ship off the coast of South America.[5]

"When I took by Storm the two Cities of Guaiaquil (Guayaquil- a city and port of Ecuador, currently the gateway to the Galapagos Island), under the Line[6], in the South Seas, it happen'd that not long before, the Plague had raged amongst them. For our better Security, therefore, and keeping our People together, we lay in their Churches, and likewise brought thither the Plunder of the Cities: We were very much annoy'd with the Smell of the dead Bodies....In less than Forty-eight Hours we had in our several Ships, one hundred and eighty men in this miserable Condition. I order'd the Surgeons to bleed them in both Arms, and to go round to them all with Command to leave them bleeding till all were blooded.... We had on board Oil and Spirit of Vitriol (sulfuric acid) sufficient, which I caused to be mixed with Water to the Acidity of a lemon, and make them drink very freely of it; so that notwithstanding we had one

---

[5] Ibid: p. 100 – 102.

[6] The Line probably refers to the line drawn by the Treaty of Zaragoza between Spain and Portugal in 1494 that divided their respective spheres of influence, those to the East belonged to Portugal and to the West to Spain

hundred and eighty odd down in this most fatal Distemper, yet we lost on more than seven or eight; **and even these owed their Deaths to the strong Liquors which their Mess-Mates procured for them."**

While as we see Thomas Dover was a believer in bleeding for anything that could be classified as inflammation, as were all the doctors in his day, he also employed quicksilver or metallic mercury with abandon. He was often called the Quicksilver doctor. He scolded his colleagues who employed blisters (application of Cantharides, Spanish flies, or other agent that would produce a blister as a counter irritant). Dover favored the introduction of inoculation against smallpox and opposed older treatments recommended by Paracelsus such as bezoar stones and other outdated nostrums.[7] He was always respectful to his teacher, Sydenham advocating relief of pain and cold baths for fever, but not mentioning horseback riding which was one of Sydenham's favorite remedies. Because Dover's doses of narcotics were considered excessive his opponents advised his patients to prepare their wills before consulting him. However Dover countered with tales of wondrous lightening-like cures, with letters from gratified patients to back up his claims for cures for everything from the gout to the dropsy. It is in this book, *The Ancient Physicians Legacy* on page 14 as the third remedy for gout, not the first, that the famous prescription for the preparation of his powder is set forth.

---

[7] Ibid: p. xxv – xxvii.

Take Opium one Ounce, Salt-Petre and Tartar vitriolated, each four Ounces Ipocacuana one Ounce, Liquorish one Ounce. Put the Salt-Petre and Tartar into a red hot Mortar, stirring when with a Spoon till they have done flaming,- Then powder them very fine; after that slice in your Opium; grind these to a Powder, and then mix the other Powders with these. Dose from forty to sixty or seventy Grains in a Glass of White-Wine Posset, going to bed.- Covering up warm, and drinking a Quart or three pints of the Posset-Drink while sweating."

Dover continues describing the expected effects of his Powder on the gout. "In two or three Hours, at farthest, the Patient will be perfectly free from Pain: and though before not able to put one Foot to the Ground, 'tis very much if he cannot walk the next Day." Thomas Dover continues commenting on criticism of others concerning the dose of Opiates, " Some Apothecaries have desired their Patients to make their Wills, and settle their Affairs, before they venture upon so large a Dose as I have recommended, which is from Forty to Seventy Grains. As monstrous as they may represent this, I can produce undeniable Proofs, where a Patient of mine has taken to no less a Quantity than an Hundred Grains, and yet has appear'd abroad the next Day." As to why this high dose is well tolerated, Dover had a suggestion, " This Notion of theirs (that a high dose is detrimental) proceeds entirely from their Ignorance, and from the Want of knowing the Nature of those Ingredients that are mix'd up with it, for they naturally weaken the Power of the Opium."

Let us examine the composition of Dover's powder more carefully. The first ingredient Opium, one Ounce was as well known and appreciated then as today. Poppy, Papaver sominiferum grown extensively in many countries of Europe and Asia as well as America, reaches a height of 2-3 feet with seeds and flowers of various colors. It is the dried seeds producing a milky extract of various alkaloids, morphine, codeine, papaverine, etc. that is obtained from the dried material. Opium has a long and well known history from Assyrian times to the Opium Wars of the 19th century, and in works of literature as well. Opium is primarily a pain reliever, blocking the opium receptors of the brain but useful in diarrhea. It was probably the major factor in the relief of Dover's patient with gout, relieving his pain "in two to three hours, at the farthest (to) be perfectly free from pain; and though before not able to put one foot to the ground, 'tis very much if he cannot walk the next day." It is doubtful if it had any direct or long lasting effect on the gout itself. In fact Dover goes on to plug "Mynsycht's Elixir of Vitriol taken in large quantities most certainly destroys gouty matter; yet for some time it may cause pain; but taken in its due latitude, if water will quench fire it must in the end have its desired effects." [8] Mynsycht's Elixir of Vitriol, Acid vitrioli aromaticaticum, is sulfuric acid in wine, introduced by Adrian Mynsycht in 1631, the formula including many other aromatics as well. Opium can produce sweating or diaphoresis by increasing peripheral blood flow.[9] Such effects

---

[8] Ibid: p.14-15.

[9] US Dispensatory, 34th edition, 1947, p. 717. On this same page Dover's powder is listed as a diaphoretic for "colds and rheumatism"

were to become the powder's chief usage. These properties were attributed to Dover's powder by later observers as well as by Dover himself. The "covering up warm, and drinking a quart or three pints of the Posset-Drink while sweating" may have been an added significant effect, as well.

Next let us consider the Salt-Petre and Tartar vitriolated, each four Ounces which I will consider as filler agents. Salt-Petre or Sal Nitre is potassium nitrate and Tartar vitriolated is Kali sulphuratum or potassium sulfate, adding some grittiness to the overall mechanical effect of the powder.

Next comes Ipocacuana, one Ounce. Ipecacuanha comes from the root of a small shrub like plant grown in Brazil. The name of the plant reflects the Portuguese native word, i-pe-kaa-guene which means "road-side sick-making plant" reflecting the ability to induce vomiting by its primary ingredient, Emetine. The chief ingredients of ipecac are the alkaloids Emetine, cephaelin and Psychotrine. 1.5 to 2% of the bark contains these alkaloids of which Emetine is the major component. At low doses ¼ to 2 grains Ipecac is an expectorant and diaphoretic but at larger doses, 15 to 20 grains, the more familiar effect of vomiting is predominant.

The next element in Dover's powder is Liquorish, one ounce. Licorice is also a root of the plant, Glycerrihiza glaba. It has a sweat taste and mildly cathartic. It is often included in Chinese herb mixtures and was known in the ancient world and grows widely. King Tutankhamen was even buried with a supply. The sweetness of the material is related to glycyrrhizic acid, a compound with two sugars attached to a steroid-like molecule. It has been known that glycyrrhizic can support patients with adrenal insufficiency, but it wasn't recognized until relatively recently that it modulates the 11 beta hydroxy-dehydrogenase, decreasing the degradation of cortisol.[10] The similarity of the structure of glycyrrhetic acid to that of steroids may also contribute to its cortisol effect.[11] Licorice finds its usage not only as a sweet agent in candy but as flavoring agents in tobacco, soft drinks, in cough syrup and in medicines to mask their bitter taste. The latter effect is the one Thomas Dover employed in his famous powder to mask the otherwise bitter mixture.

And what about the White wine Posset ? A Posset is milk curdled with beer, wine or other liquor. A typical Posset is a mixture of 2 parts small beer and one part milk. Undoubtedly the alcohol was a contributing factor to the salutary effect experienced with Dover's patient in gout.

---

[10] Whorwood, C.B., Sheppard, M.C., Stewart, P.M. Licorice inhibits 11beta-hydroxysteroid dehydrogenase messenger ribonucleic acid levels and potentiates glucocorticoid hormone action. Endocrinology June, 132(6) 1993. p.2287-2287. As a Resident in Medicine in 1954, I took care of a patient with a bilateral subtotal adrenalectomy, performed for severe hypertension. He had taken steroid replacement irregularly but had been taking large doses of licorice. This habit aggravated his parents who took the licorice from him, hiding the material to break his habit of excessive licorice ingestion. He promptly went into Adrenal insufficiency but was stabilized with saline and Cortisol. At the time the licorice was considered to contain a steroid like substance that directly replaced the missing Cortisol.

[11] Armanini, D, Karbowiak I, Funder JW, Affinity of liquorice derivatives for mineralocorticoid and glucocorticoid receptors, Clin Endocrinol (Oxf) 19, 609-612, 1983.

The major ingredients in Dover's powder are opium and ipecac. One ounce of each or 30 grams in a total of 11 ounces or 330 grams of the entire mixture. Let us consider the opium first and making some assumptions such as the amount of the active ingredient morphine being about 10 % of the total opium. Now noting Dover's prescription of a "dose from forty to sixty to seventy grains in a glass of white-wine posset, going to bed" it is calculated that about 0.36 grains (5.40 mg) of morphine to be present in the forty grain dosage and that in the seventy grain dose would contain 0.63 grains (9.5 mg) morphine. Opium contains additional alkaloids other than morphine that might increase its potency, but taking the mixture orally would reduce its immediate effectiveness. Certainly a potent dose of a narcotic, but not an excessive dose of opium that would hardly warrant his opponents recommending that the recipients write out their wills before taking Dover's powder. The same sort of assumptions can apply to the ipecacuanha root. The 40 grain dose would contain about 3.6 grains of ipecac and the 70 grain dose about 6.3 grains of ipecac. Both of these dosages would contain what is considered a low dose, 0.25 to 2.0 grains enough to result in sweating or expectoration. Larger doses of 15 to 30 grains have the more familiar emetic function.

One of the striking features of this Dover's Powder is the absence of a single potent cathartic in the mixture, which was usually present in the nostrums of the day. I considered that double dose of potassium containing drugs, Salt Petre (potassium nitrate) and Tartar Vitrioated (potassium sulfate) might lead to potassium intoxication, but calculation suggests that it was not an excessive amount. The avoidance of a high dose of ipecac, minimizing vomiting but promoting the sudorific aspects of the mixture, was either a point of pharmacological insight or a piece of good luck. The opium and the ipecac acted in concert to produce this effect as a sweating agent, so important in the later use of the powder. It was probably serendipity that combined a low dose of ipecac and a hefty dose of opium, at least enough to cure the patient's acute gouty distemper, rather than have to experiment with a controlled drug trial. And how about that parting touch with the use of that sweet Liquorish to make the powder palatable? Its bitterness without the Liquorish might not have sold so well. It adds up to a masterful stroke for patients and the medical profession.

The preparation of Dover's powder is rather challenging for anyone, including an apothecary. The salt-petre and tartar vitriolated are "put into a red-hot mortar, stirring them with a spoon till they have done flaming, then powdered fine." How many homes then or today have that "red hot mortar" available? Then the opium is sliced in, ground to a powder and then mixed with the other powder. Even our contemporary pharmacist might struggle with its preparation, especially arranging for that "red hot mortar" and all that "stirring with a spoon till they have done flaming" and grinding to a powder, shaving and mixing. Certainly this is not the usual off the shelf prescription we are accustomed to see our pharmacists prepare.

Dower was certainly very familiar with the clinical presentation of gout for which his powder was to alleviate. The following extended description may serve to remind contemporary physicians what gout was like in the early eighteenth century.

A regular gout may most properly be term'd Podagra, because it begins in the first joint of the great toe, and usually about midnight; where, after it has rack'd the patient forty-eight hours with a violent fixed pain, a small tumour begins to appear, increasing gradually; after that, an inflammation, and then the violence of the pain abates.

The first fit may last a fortnight, or three weeks; but a great weakness and tenderness in the part afflicted, remains much longer.

The patient may feel no more of this disease for two or three years, or at soonest a twelvemonth: but what adds much to the misfortune of this distemper, is, that every fit becomes more painful, and the paroxysms more frequent and lasting.

The gouty matter increasing, rises to the ankles and knees, which, as was said before, swell with inflammation: This degree of the distemper, by some authors is called Morbus Articularis, and is always attended with asymptomatical fever; for as the pain wears off, the fever abates.

Thus it takes its progress, increasing by degrees, till the poor patient is lacerated, and torn to pieces; chalk-stones working out of the joints, attended with other melancholy circumstances.

It must be observed, towards the latter end of this disease, when the fluids are almost wholly changed into gouty matter, the fits are not so regular, nor the pains so violent; but then the patient is seldom free from them.[12]

Thomas Dower's description of diseases in his *Physician's Legacy to his Country* is usually not as vividly drawn, but his familiarity with gout, as well as compassion toward the patient is apparent in this description. He goes on to consider therapy. "There have been so many unsuccessful attempt made to alter this disease, that patients have very little faith left, and (as they commonly say) have no hopes from any thing but patience and warm flannel....Notwithstanding the many fruitless attempts that have been made to cure this miserable distemper, providence has in this, as well as in all other diseases, left means for recovery, which in many instances I am able to make appear."[13] His confidence and braggadocio make their appearance here. "I shall refer to one (cure), where the curious may be satisfied: The coachman of the right honourable the Lord Viscount St. John had a long and tedious fit of the gout, and was hardly able to stir without crutches; I gave him a very pleasant easy Sudorific (not further characterized); which had its desired effect: - Insomuch that the day following, he walked from Albemarle-street to Cecil-street, to give me thanks. He came to me without the help of a stick and with strait shoes on: the swelling was entirely gone: he affirmed that he was never better in his life; and that he as able to walk from one end of the town to

---

[12] Dewhust, Kenneth, facsimile edition of The Ancient Physician's Legacy, 1947, p.9-10.

[13] Ibid, p. 11.

the other. This is about twenty–five Years ago."[14]
Now this was an appreciative patient!

That "pleasant easy Sudorific" not further
characterized was the first prescription
recommended for the gout by Dover. The second
prescription "without Opiates, or painful remedies
which I am a stranger to and very much dislike"
follows:

Take **Tamarinds** *half an ounce, leaves of* **Senna** *two
drams,* **Rheuberb** *one dram, boil them in water to
three ounces; strain them off, and dissove in them of*
manna *and the purging syrup of roses, each one ounce
syrup of* **buck-thorn** *and* **Elixer Proprietatis***, each two
drams. – Drinking* **Posset-Drink***, or thin gruel between
motion, - taking this once or twice a week will lessen the
gouty matter, and break the force of the fit.*[15]

Tamarinds is a large tree from India with multiple
alleged pharmacological usages including as a
cathartic. **Senna** is a small shrub. The name is
Arabian and its leaves are known for purgative
action. The tea is popular today. **Rheuberb** also a
mild cathartic from the root of a common garden
plant. **Manna,** probably not the manna or bread
from the bible but the resin from *Fraxinus ornus*, is
again a weak cathartic from which mannose and
mannital were first isolated. **Buckthorn,** has berries
that are a strong cathartic. **Elixer Proprietatis**
(Paracelsi) referring to Paracelsus's own elixir, from
the inspissated juice of aloe, from Arabian sea, used
as a cathartic today.

---

[14] Ibid. p.12.

[15] Ibid p.13.

While Dover recommends that "taking this once or twice a week, will lessen the gouty matter and break the force of the fits", it is certainly plainly evident that this fourth prescription for gout is nothing but a mixture of laxatives having this as its primary purpose.

It was the third prescription of Thomas Dover to improve gout, **Pulvis Ipecacunanhae et Opii** that remained in the Pharmacopoeia for over 200 years. Its unique combination of opium and ipecac became popular as a diaphoretic agent and later, as with William Osler, as an agent for relief of diarrhea along with a host of other presumed usages. Kenneth Dewhurst in his *Thomas Dover's Life and Legacy,* indicates that "After Dover's death it (the powder) was appropriated by the quack Joshua Ward who popularized it as a sweating powder. After Wards death his recipe book was found to contain details of two powders, one identical with Dover's recipe, and the other with the addition of white hellebore (root of the white hellebore, *Veratrum viride,* an emetic containing several alkaloids). This plagiarism probably saved Dover's powder from passing into obscurity, and certainly led to its inclusion in the London Pharmacopoeia of 1788."[16] This was forty six years after his heath in 1735 and fifty six years after the publication of the first edition of the *Ancient Physician's legacy to his Country* in 1732. Dover probably would have been surprised by the acclaim later generation would apply to his powder, since during his life time his use of mercury was his

---

[16] Dewhurst, Kenneth, Thomas Dover's Life and Legacy, published under the auspices of the Library of the New York Academy of Medicine, The Scarecrow Press, Inc, Metuchen , N.J. 1974, p.xxvii.

defining attribute, since he was known as the "quicksilver doctor."

Roy Porter in his *The Greatest Benefits to Mankind* in his chapter on the Enlightenment indicates that " The eighteenth century has been dubbed the golden age of quackery (an obscure term that may have come from the Dutch 'quacksalver' or quicksilver doctor)."[17]   Quacks included such people as Mesmer, with his magnets, James Grahman a Scot who advocated mud bathing and the electrified Celestial Bed, as well as Joshua Ward (1685-1761). He made a fortune out of his "pill and drop", antimony, an antipyretic and an emetic and the "drop" being a vigorous purgative having multiple effects, as well as his recipe book perpetuating Dover's powder as a sweating agent.

Dover's Powder was well received by the community of physicians. While its use as an agent in gout was disappointing, its use as a depletion therapy, especially to encourage sweating, took hold. "The age-old medical regimes: blood-letting, sweating, purging, vomiting and other ways of expelling bad humours had a hold upon the popular imagination and reflected medical confidence in such matters."[18]   J. Worth Estes in *Hospital Life in Enlightenment Scotland* traces Dr. Andrew Duncan's, Sr. attendance and use of

---

[17] Porter Roy, Greatest Benefit to Mankind, W.W. Norton and Company, New York/London, 1997, p.284-285.

[18] Ibid: p.674.

medication on the teaching ward of the Royal Infirmary of Edinburgh in 1795.[19]

Phyllis V. age 42 was admitted to the infirmary with a diagnosis of diabetes mellitus with polydipsia, polyphagia, and massive polyuria. Initally the patient was treated with **alum** to decrease excessive urine output, then **Cinchona,** presumably for the same reason, **blistering,** on day 15. **An emetic** and a **cathartic** to strengthen the patient's stomach and relax her bowels. Since the urine output remained high, **cold water compresses** were applied over the kidneys followed by electricity over the kidneys. "She was still spilling excess sugar into her urine, as determined by tasting it!" She then developed signs of a respiratory infection and was treated with similar agents. " He also prescribed **Dover's powder** as a diaphoretic to help remove the fever." After additional treatments including dilute solution of **cantharides** orally, lime water, urine out put stabilized at less that five pounds per day (2400 ml) and after six months in the hospital she was discharged.

The difficulties of treating diabetes before insulin are apparent and Dover's powder became one of the mélange of medications commonly used at that period.

Richard Bright at Guy's Hospital in London, reported in 1827 on the triad of dropsy, coagulable urine and abnormal granular kidneys. While his list of medications include many of the agents popular

---

[19] Risse, Guenter B, Hospital life in Enlightenment Scotland, Appendix D, Drug usage at the infirmary: the example of Dr. Andrew Duncan, Sr., by J Worth Estes, p.361 – 364.

in the day, similar to those at the Royal Infirmary of Edinburgh, from where he received his medical degree, Dower's powder was not one of his favorite choices. However Case 1, John King did received some of the components: Sumat Mist. effervese. cum **Vini Ipecacuanhae**, Olei Ricini cum **Tinct. Opii.** The ipecac, and opium are there as well as caster oil, but not according to the specifications of Dover.

A more enthusiastic proponent would be Johnathan Osborne of Dublin who following the lead of Bright confirmed much of his findings in a slim volume entitled *On the Nature and Treatment of Dropsical Diseases*, 1833. He was much impressed by the finding of "suppressed perspiration" as a major cause of this form of renal disease. He vigorously employed warm baths of every source, along with Dover's powder, reporting remarkable improvement in patient's general condition. "When a patient was placed under my care with general edema coagulable urine and dry skin, I direct him to be kept in bed, in order to maintain warmth of the surface...The first medication is a purgative followed by a foot bath, hip bath, or general bath, water or vapor at night with *Pulvi Ipeac with Opio.*"[20] Four of his six reported cases received warm baths and *Pulvi. Doveri.*

Another follower of Richard Bright was Robert Christian of Edinburgh who likewise confirmed Bright's observation and in 1829 and 1839 and declared, " the most efficient diaphoretic is Dover's

---

[20] Osborne, Jonathan, On the Nature and Treatment of Dropsical Diseases, 1833, p.76.

powder with a warm bath." He employed the powder in the management of many of his cases.

No one can question the propriety of the diaphoretic method of cure of the primary disease.The most efficient diaphoretic is **Dover's powder** which should always be conjoined with the warm bath. No other remedy gives more relief...so that its ultimate good effects can be scarcely be doubted. It commonly occasions sweating for some time afterwards and is followed by quiet sleep. **Dover's powder** is preferable to (Acetate of ammonium) being scarcely less useful as an anodyne and calmitive for removing pain and allaying irritability and restlessness. [21]

Such were the accolades provided by Robert Christian for the treatment of granular degeneration, his name for the condition described by Bright several years earlier. Note how Dover's Powder is praised as an complement to warm baths as a diaphoretic agent, but also by virtue of it containing opium, as calming and analgesic agent, reinforcing the original use of the powder as a treatment for gout. And yet of the thirty one cases presented by Christian only five received the powder. This may be explained by Christian's later reservation about the enthusiastic results of Osborne. " I sincerely wish that my experience of the effects of the diaphoretic plan could bear out the very sanguine encomiums bestowed upon it by Dr. Osborne.... I have several time seen general perspiration both spontaneous and from the use of diaphoretics fail to produce any material relief.

[21] Christian, Robert, On Granular Degeneration of the Kidnies and its Connection with Dropsy, Inflammations and other Diseases, 1939, p. 65.

Still no one can question the general propriety of the diphoretic method of cure. "[22]

On the other hand, Pierre Rayer considered the founder of French Nephrology, while recommending warm baths and perspiration, eschewed the use of Dover's powder. In his *Traite des Maladies des Reins et des Alterations de la Secretion Urinaire*[23] while favoring wild horseradish tea as a diuretic, and recommending warm baths, the "English Pathologists" recommendation for Dover's powder comes in for some rebuke.

"A few successes resulting from steam baths in the treatment of this dropsy have naturally led to trying diaphoretics and several agents which have a remarkable influence on the functioning of the skin. The well-known relationship between the functions of the skin and the urinary functions seem to fortify the hopes that are most rarely realized.

English pathologists generally recommend Dover's powder, repeated three times a day as a powerful diaphoretic. James Powder (Antimony calcium phosphate) *passes among them for a good diaphoretic; for my part, I feel myself obliged to declare that the trials I have made with these remedies in the treatment of dropsy stemming from chronic albuminous nephritis, have been almost completely unfruitful; rarely have these powders induced a salutary perspiration and often the Dower's powder has been the occasion of malaise and the*

---

[22] Ibid: p. 65-66.

[23] Rayer, Pierre, Traite des Maladies des Reins et des Alterations de la Secretion Urinaire, 1840. p.152-153. (Translation by T Carr and R.I.Levy, to be published)

desire to vomit. The diaphoresis, that these remedies have produced in some cases, has had no or almost no advantageous influence on the progress of the dropsy.

Rayer may not have incorporated Dover's balanced mixture of opium and ipecac, as originally recommended, avoiding the emetic effect of the later and the "malaise" of the former. He was very familiar with the reports of Bright, as well with the studies of Jonathan Osborne in Ireland on the effect of perspiration induced with baths and Dover's powder   At this point Rayer commenting on Jonathan Osborne in *On dropsies connected with suppressed perspiration and coagulable urine, London, 18 35,* "Doctor Osborne is said to have cured 27 patients out of 36 (remarkable result if, among these cases, there were not a lot of acute cases), following a method which is in reality only the joining of the most recommended of means (blood letting, cupping glasses, purgatives, simple baths, steam baths, sudorifics, vesicatories, etc.) but what he uses with a particular view in mind, that of reestablishing cutaneous perspiration which (he believes) is almost always suppressed in this disease. Dr. Osborne explains the salutary effects of these remedies, of bleeding, even of vesicatories, by diaphoresis." [24]   Here Rayer seems to cast doubt on the   results of Osborne as well as on the effectiveness of sweating, as applied to Dover's powder in the ability to modify the underlying disease process.

SUMMARY

------

[24] Ibid: p.153 footnote.

Thomas Dover followed his apprenticeship with Sydenham with a tour of duty as a sea captain before settling down to the practice of medicine. His swashbuckling style flavored his medical writing in his *The Ancient Physician's Legacy to his Country*, with tales of adventure as "when (he) took by storm the two Cities of Guaiaquil" during the plague epidemic. While respectful of the teachings of his mentor, Sydenham, favoring cold baths and comforting the patient, he was equally vehement in deprecating those who followed the older methods of Paracelsus or advocated blistering. "An eminent Physician was ask'd, How Blistering came so much in Fashion? He answer'd they had it from the Indians. But I, that have seen more Indians than all the Physicians in England deny that the Indians ever make use of Blisters. They do often cauterize; and in all Fevers amongst them, they cover the Patients over in the Sand till they are in profuse Sweat, and then throw them into cold Water; by which Means they become well."[25] The use of cold water may be a tribute to his mentor, Sydenham.

Dover's powder, his third attempt to cure gout, became his one claim to immortality with his buccaneering exploits in the background. Wonderfully designed to contain just the right dose of opium to give relief from pain and providing some diaphoretic effect, it avoided a high dose of ipecac that would have produced vomiting yet preserving its alleged diaphoretic action (Rayer's experience with the Powder causing vomiting and malaise to the contrary). The Powder was tastefully

---

[25] Dewhurst, Kenneth, *Thomas Dover's Life and Legacy*, facsimile edition of *The Ancient Physician's Legacy to his Country*, p 105.

seasoned with a dash of Liquorish to mask the bitter taste, combined with fillers to improve the mechanical feel of the powder. The preparation went on to be serviceable as a diaphoretic and as with many other medication, to have alternative or off-label uses as well. The dose of Opium was always welcome as an analgesic or to counter diarrhea as with William Osler almost two hundred years later. Of course the white Poset wine used as a chaser in the original prescription for gout was a nice touch. But was Dover's powder alone really that effective as a diaphoretic or was it all those warm baths and heavy blankets and white wine Posset that did the trick? Was Pierre Rayer's condemnation of Dover's powder just a proud Frenchman's rebuttal to the "English pathologist" or were his observations cogent?

Chapter Five

William Harvey's *De Motu Cordis and the Heart as Metaphor*

"When first I applied my mind to observation from the many dissections of Living Creatures , that I might find out the use of the motion of the Heart; I straightwayes found it a thing hard to be attained, and full of difficulty, so with **Fracastorius** *I did almost believe that the motion of the Heart was known to God alone.* [1]

William Harvey, Chapter 1, **De Motu Cordis**

Introduction: Heart as Metaphor

Following the publication of William Harvey's **De Motu Cordis** (The Motion of the Heart) in 1628, the physiology of the heart and the circulation, initially accepted by very few, slowly became almost universally accepted in Harvey's lifetime.

---

[1]. Willis, R. William Harvey, A History of the Discovery of the Circulation of the Blood, 1878. In a footnote on p. 186 Willis refers to Fracastorius' *Opera Omnia* where he considered the purpose of "attraction of air and the fuliginous vapours" being known only to God, rather than the motion of the heart as stated by Harvey.

Prior to that time the function of the heart was considered in numerous ways and so translated into our language with many expressions that mirrored these speculations. " The heart, that most 'noble' of organs, was seen variously as a center of heat, life, or emotional force. Not until the seventeenth century did William Harvey lower it's kingly status to more or less that of a lowly pump."[2] The myriad metaphors in our language regarding the heart reflect the history of what was thought to be its function. Thus both Aristotle and Galen considered that an important function of the heart was to provide innate heat.[3] This is probably the origin of the expression *a warm hearted person*, still present in our language. From the Hebrew bible comes the commandment, " *Thou shalt love the Lord thy God with all thy **heart** and with all thy **soul** - and these words, which I command thee this day, shall be inscribed in thine **heart**."*[4] The second **heart** in this biblical expression brings to mind the expression to **learn something by heart.** Here we see the brain, considered much less important than the heart in ancient days, taking second place to the heart for memory. The Hebrew bible uses the word **Heart** (*lev*) over 850 times, sometimes associated with the kidney as well. [5] William Harvey's *De Motu Cordis* clarified the physiological role of the heart as a pump to

---

[2] Rather, L. J. , Metaphorical Language in the History of Western Medicine, A celebration of Medical History, Baltimore: Johns Hopkins University Press, 1982, p. 138.

[3] May, T. M. Galen – On the Usefulness of the Parts of the Body, Introduction Galen's System of Physiology, p. 50.

[4] Deuteronomy, VI: 5-6.

[5] Hoystad, Ole, A History of the Heart,p.58. Reaktion Books Ltd, London 2007.

circulate the blood, ending these speculative functions of the heart. Our language is continually enriched by the use of these notions of the heart's function which we continue to use , in spite of its true physiological function.

In Shakespeare's Concordance there are listed 1047 references to the heart, many metaphorical. What did Iago in Othello mean by, " I will wear my *Heart* on my sleeve? The Oxford English Dictionary lists 53 pages of the these different meanings of the word "heart."

Such metaphoric uses of the heart are almost daily occurrence in newspapers and speech.

A Heartfelt homecoming
Speak from the Heart
Playing by Heart

Galen's Description of the Heart

In first considering the problem of the heart, William Harvey (1578–1657) would have considered the ancient teachings of Galen, which represented the medical, anatomical, and physiological function of the body for fourteen hundred years. Galen was grounded in the anatomy mostly of animals, since dissection of human cadavers was forbidden. Arteries were considered to contain air, from which arteries as well as the aorta were named, but one of Galen's great achievements was to prove that this was not the case.[6] He placed a ligature in two places about

---

[6] Erasistratus in the 2nd century BC had claimed the arteries contained air

an artery, incised the artery between the ligatures and found no air but only blood. Another experiment of Galen on the nervous system address the relative roles of the heart or brain in the production of speech. "Galen's experimental proof that it is the brain and not the heart that controls the voice was proven by Galen by cutting the recurrent laryngeal nerve, which he knew came from the brain and not the heart, producing a dramatic loss of the voice in a squealing pig that was his subject. He also had the opportunity to observe the same loss of voice in two men whose laryngeal nerve was accidentally severed by physicians. "[7]

These careful experiments in physiology contrast with Galen's fanciful description of the heart and its function that was to represent the established doctrine of Western Medicine for fourteen centuries, which would be finally overturned in 1628 by Harvey's *De Motu Cordis:*

Venous blood was elaborated in the liver traveled to the upper and lower parts of the body.

Venous and arterial blood were contained in separate vessels and were in constant oscillatory motion, to nourish the limbs. Arterial blood was "spiritualized" by the air from the lungs, moderating the heat of the left ventricle and providing a source of vitality.

The heart attracted the blood in diastole or dilation, like a magnet attracts iron. The diastole was the

---

[7] Ibid p.63

active "aspiration" of the cardiac walls and the systole the passive relapsing of the walls.

Galen convinced himself of the presence of pores or foramina in the intraventricular septum. [8]

Sixteenth Century's Reconsideration of Heart Function—Prelude to William Harvey

In the 16th century Michael Servetus, physician and theologian, dared to suggest a pulmonary circulation and denied a communication between the septum, in his book, *Restitution of Christianity* (1533), but his theological arguments were considered heretical by Calvin and he was burned at the stake along with almost all his books.[9] Leonardo da Vinci in the latter part of the sixteenth century made remarkably accurate drawings of the human heart, its valves and blood vessels, but never denied the presence of pores in the cardiac septum. Realdus Columbo, an assistant to Vesalius, considered a pulmonary transit, finding blood, instead of air in the pulmonary vein as indicated by Galen.[10] He also indicated that there were no pores in the ventricular septum and that the valves of the heart were competent preventing blood from returning to the lungs. [11]Andreas Caesalpinus also considered a pulmonary

---

[8] Chauvois, Louis, William Harvey, His Life and Times: His Discoveries: His Methods, Philosophical Library,p.183-186.

[9] Osler, William, Michael Servetus, Johns Hopkins Hospital Buletin, xxi., 1910, p. 1-11.

[10] Whitteridge, G., William Harvey and the Circulation of the Blood, 1971, p41 – 59.

[11] Ibid. p. 53.

circulation.[12] Hieromymus Fabricius, Harvey's teacher at Padua, described the valves in the veins in 1603 in his *Venarium Ostiolis.*[13] Nevertheless, the views of Galen on the separation of the venous and arterial systems, the to and fro nature of the blood flow, and presence of pores in the ventricular wall all remained the gospel according to Galen until William Harvey's 1628 *De Motu Cordis.*

William Harvey—Early Life, Medical School at Padua and Return to England

William Harvey was born in the little town of Folkestone on the southeastern coast of England in Kent during the reign of Elizabeth I in April 1578. After he attended Caius College at Cambridge University, he then traveled to the University of Padua in Italy in 1600 to complete medical studies under Fabricius.[14] Harvey returned to England in 1602 to practice medicine. He was appointed to St. Bartholomew's Hospital in London , later becoming a member of the prestigious College of Physicians and eventually becoming physician to two kings of England, James I and Charles I as well as to ponder the possibility of the circulation of blood.

Harvey's Interest in Rethinking Function the of the Heart—The Prelectiones and De Motu Cordis

---

[12] Pagel, W., William Harvey's Biological Ideas, 1967, p. 171.

[13] Bylerbly, Jerome, The Medical Side of Harvey's Discovery, p. 60-61, WilliamHarvey and His Age, Edited by Jerome J. Bylebyl. Johns Hopkins Press, 1979.

[14] Keynes, Geoffrey, The Life of William Harvey , p.26, Oxford at the Clarendon Press, 1978

In 1616 Harvey was appointed to the important post of Lumleian Lecturer. These lectures had been founded by John Lumley in 1582 to "raise the repute of both surgery and anatomy" and were given at two year intervals.[15] Harvey's lecture notes, or *Praelectiones* , were anatomical exercises but indicate his increasing interest in experimentation on the hearts of cold blooded animals, such as snakes , frogs, eels, and fish, where the pulse rate allowed more accurate demonstration of the action of the heart beat. In these Anatomical Lectures from 1616, Harvey writes, "*When the heart is relaxed, which happens first, there is an entering into it of blood into the right ventricle from the vena cava, and into the left (ventricle) from the pulmonary vein. When it is erected or contracted it drives out the blood as it were by force from the right ventricle into the lungs and from the left ventricle into the aorta, and this is the reason for the arterial pulse.*"[16] Galen had considered that the arterial pulse was generated by the contraction of the arterial wall itself , synchronous with the contraction of the heart.[17]

Thus early on Harvey emphasized an important correction to Galen's doctrine that diastole was the active function of the cardiac action, drawing the blood into its chamber. In these Lectures, "*Harvey looked to the heartbeat, and more particularly to the powerful contractions of the heart in systole , as the*

---

[15] Ibid., p.86.

[16] Whitteridge, Gweneth, The anatomical Lectures of William Harvey, Published for the Royal College of Physicians , London, by E and S. Livingstone Ltd, Edinburgh and London, p. 271-273, 1971.

[17] Ibid. p. 45.

crucial biological activity whose primary purpose is to continually force blood outward through the arteries to all parts of the body."[18]   These are essentially the arguments made for the heart's function in De Motu Cordis, chapter 2 and the early chapters, with the concept of the circulation as a natural extension occupying the second half of the book, all published twelve years later when he was fifty years old, in 1628.[19]

Quantitative Method to Support the Concept of the Circulation of the Blood

To support his concept of the circulation of the blood, Harvey in chapter 9 of *De Motu Cordis* makes use of a quantitative method. Galen had postulated that the liver transferred ingested food as the origin and motion of the blood.[20] Harvey then presented a quantitative argument where cardiac output was only estimated, and these assumptions were low. Harvey then considered in one hour there would be 2000 heart beats. This figure is also low, 33 beats per minute, leading us to questioning whether Harvey used a watch !

---

[18] Bylebyl, Jerome, William Harvey and His Age p. 68

[19] Bylebyl, Jerome, The Growth of Harvey's De Motu Cordis, p. 449, p. 451, "Originally, Harvey seems to have written a self-contained treatise on the heartbeat and arterial pulse. Subsequently he changed his plans and decided to include the circulation as well."

[20] Kilgour, Frederick, C., William Harvey's Use of the Quantitative Method, Presented before the Beaumont Club, 3/14/1952

Harvey did indeed have a time piece, a watch with a minute hand according to John Aubrey in *Brief Lives* , a biography of prominent men in seventeenth century England. Aubrey indicates that near death, Harvey gave *"to one of his nephews a watch with a minute hand with which he made his experiments."* [21] Even using these low, inaccurate estimates the cardiac output would represent an enormous amount of blood, 180 liters just in one hour, which could not be possible from Galen's theory of blood production in the liver from food.[22] Harvey didn't need exact quantities of cardiac output or even a more accurate measure of pulse rate. More accurate measurements would not have altered his conclusion that the only way such a large volume of blood ejected from the heart could be produced was by the concept of a circulation.[23]

Quantitative methods as applied to biology or medicine were unusual but were performed in the early 17th century. Galileo, Santorio, and Van Helmont all performed quantitative studies with more accurate data.

Additional Studies to Support the Concept of the Circulation of the Blood

---

[21] Aubrey, John, Aubrey's Brief Lives, London, Secker and Warburg, 1949, p. 132. Watches in the first part of the 17th century were spring watches which were not great time keepers. C. Huygens in 1675 inventor the spiral spring balance which improved their reliability. Heilbrunn Time line 17th Century watches.

[22] Cardiac output = Heart rate X Stroke volume   72/min X 70 ml = 5 liters/min or 300 liters/one hour

[23] Kilgour, Frederick, William Harvey's use of the Quantitative Method, Presented before the Beaumont Club, 3/14/1952, modified after Frederick Kilgour, p. 416 - 418

In the following chapters of his book, Harvey describes experiments with ligatures applied to the limbs that support the proposition that blood passes from the arteries into the veins. In Fig. 1 of this well known engraved plate a loose ligature, as applied in blood letting. In Fig. 2 "drawing the blood down from O to H", the valve at O prevents blood flowing distally, allowing only for blood flow centrally to the heart. These two engraved plates were not original but redrawn after that previously published by Fabricius, which was the first adequate illustration of the valves of the veins. [24]

Robert Boyle, chemist and one of the founders of the Royal Society, recalls questioning Harvey as to what had induced him to consider the circulation of the blood. Harvey pointed to the valves in the veins, discovered by Fabricius who considered they only regulated the to and fro flow. Harvey, however, interpreted the function of these valves differently, emphasizing their function as preventing the peripheral flow of blood to the extremities, giving free passage of the blood to return to the heart. [25]

Of course Harvey had no direct evidence for the passage of blood from artery to vein which was not proven until 1661 with Marcello Malpighi's

---

[24] Keynes, Geoffrey, The Life of William Harvey Oxford Press, 1978, p. 177.

[25] Boyle, R., A Disquisition about the final Causes of Natural Things, p.157, 1688. As quoted by Keynes,G. in The Life of William Harvey, p.28.

description of capillaries in the lung and of its later confirmation by Leeuenhoek.

Publication of De Motu Cordis

William Harvey' s book, *De Motu Cordis,* was published in Frankfort, Germany, in 1628. Harvey chose William Fitzer, an Englishman who had recently become a publisher and whose coat of arms appears on the title page of *De Motu Cordis.* [26] Why would an English physician choose Frankfort, Germany to publish his book? Frankfort was the site of a considerable number of printing houses as well as book fairs and Harvey thought the book could get better press and notoriety if printed in Frankfort. In addition the price of printing was less. However, the distance from England to Frankfort and the difficulty of deciphering Harvey's illegible handwriting resulted in considerable mistakes requiring an *errata leaf* of 126 items inserted in the first edition. In addition the attempt to be frugal in the printing of the book resulted in poor quality of the pages crumbling with time. [27] When I examined a first edition I was impressed by the small size of the book, 7 X 5 ¼ inches, 72 thin pages in all. William Osler gave to the Hopkins Medical School in 1906 a first edition in which is inscribed a handwritten note describing that he " had the leaf of errata taken out to insert in my copy." Osler was referring to another first edition of Harvey's book that he had previously given to McGill, which now contains the errata leaf from the Hopkins

---

[26] Keynes, Geoffrey, The Life of William Harvey, Oxford at the ClarendonPress, 1978, p. 176

[27] Ibid. p. 177

copy. The errata leaf , I have learned, is even more valuable than the original 1628 edition.

Reception of Harvey's De Motu Cordis

Initially very few of Harvey's colleagues accepted Harvey's views on the function of the heart and the concept of circulation of blood. The French were particularly intransigent. Jean Riolan, Regius Professor in Paris, very much in the mode of Galenic thinking about the heart and circulation, had numerous objections to Harvey's revolutionary ideas. This prompted Harvey to submit two letters answering Riolan's clinging Galenic belief in the pores in the septum of the heart and direction of venous flow.

Moliere in *Le Malade Imaginaire, from 1673* provides a more amusing jab at Riolan's attachment to Galenic principles. Moliere, a physician, playwright, and actor who incidentally died on stage in this play, relates the conversation between Diafoirus, a doctor – trying to praise his son, Thomas, somewhat slow witted, but in love with Angelique:

Diafoirus: " Sir, what pleases me most about him , and in this he follows my own example, in his blind attachment to the opinions of ancient authorities and his refusal ever to try to understand or even listen to the argument in favour of such *so called discoveries of our own age as the circulation of the blood and other notions of similar ilk.*"

Thomas : (taking a great scroll from his pocket and presenting it to Angelique): I have written a thesis against the *Circulationists* which--- I venture to offer to the young lady as a tribute laid before her of the first fruits of my genius."[28]

William Osler relates in his Harveian Lecture of 1906, "The satire of Moliere completed   the discomfiture of the "anticirculateurs."[29]

Discussion: Metaphors

William Harvey was not adverse to using "heart" as a metaphor in his *De Motu Cordis*. In his dedication to the King, *"Most gracious King, accept these new things concerning the (1) **Heart**, (you) who are the new light of his age, and __indeed the whole (2) Heart of it...__"* Here the first use of   Heart represents the subject of his book and the second Heart is a metaphor for the King who is the center of his age.

Harvey uses two further metaphorical references to the heart as the center, describing the King as *"the Heart of his commonwealth"* and the *"Sun, as the Heart of the world."*

In addition, in a letter Harvey writes,"I cannot find it **in my heart**, to say anything severe of Riolan"[30]

---

[28] Moliere, Le Malade Imaginaire, Act 2, scene 5.

[29] Osler,William, The Growth of Truth, As Illustrated in the Discovery of the Circulation of the Blood. Delivered before the Royal College of Physicians of London, Oct. 18 1906. Lancet Oct 26, 1906, p 1119.

[30] William Harvey and the Circulation of the Blood, Whitteridge, Gweneth,   p. 175. The letter was to Paul Marquand Slegel in 1651

Metaphors relating to the heart are a continuing everyday experience. Their origins reflect ideas from the history of the multiple functions attributable to the heart prior to William Harvey's De *Motu Cordis,* appearing frequently today in newspapers, literature, and speech.

Descartes

Descartes was one of the first to champion Harvey's theory of the circulation since it complemented his theory of a mechanical world view.[31] Harvey carefully avoided using the word *pump* to describe the heart's action in *De Motu Cordis,* substituting force out, drive out, or send forth, stressing its innate animistic force, as considered by Aristotle. Descartes in his *Discourse on Method* used Harvey's description of cardiac function to support his views of nature as mechanical and clock-like[32], while praising Harvey's discovery.

William Osler in his Harveian Lecture considered that, "The *De Motu Cordis* marked the break of the modern spirit with the old traditions."[33]

Summary

---

[31] Wright, Thomas, Circulation – William Harvey's Revolutionary Idea, Chatto and Windus, London, 2012, Essay 8, Descartes' clock work universe.

[32] Descartes, Rene, Discourse on Method, 1637, p. 65 – 72.

[33] Osler, William, The Harverian Oration of 1906, The Growth of Truth as Illustrated in the Discovery of the Circulation of the Blood, Lancet, October 27, 1906. Osler was referring to Gui Patin, dean of the Paris Medical School, very much devoted to Galen who considered the new doctrine ridiculous in allusion to the Latin word circulator, meaning charlatan.

Metaphors using the heart are discussed

Galen's vision of the heart reviewed

16th century reconsideration of fifteen centuries of Galen's concepts of the heart: Servetus, Columbo, Caesalpinus, and Fabricius.

Harvey's rethinking of the heart's function as noted in his lecture notes of 1618

Quantitative method to support the theory of the circulation discussed

Publication and reception of De Motu Cordis: Riolan, Descartes, Moliere

Absence of the Pump metaphor—Influence of Aristotle

Chapter Six

Homer W. Smith 1895-1962
Renal Physiologist

*"What is man, when you come to think upon him, but a
minutely set, ingenious machine for turning, with
Infinite artfulness, the red wine of Shiraz into urine?*[1]

Isak Dinesen, "The Dreamer"

Introduction

Homer William Smith, a Professor of Physiology at
New York University, was a dominant influence on
the developing field of renal physiology during the
first half of the twentieth century. He was
instrumental in developing the use of Inulin
clearance as a measure of glomerular filtration rate.
He wrote over 150 published articles on renal
physiology and related topics. Early studies

---

[1] Isak Dinesen, *Seven Gothic Tales*, as speculated by an Arab
sailing along the coast of Africa, quoted in Homer William
Smith, Sc.D. His Scientific and Literary Achievements, edited
by Herbert Chaisis, and William Goldring 1965, p. 127.

included those on camels, lung fish and the history of the evolution of the functional architecture of the kidney over geological time. His laboratory was a training ground for many clinicians and laboratory scientists such as William Goldring, Herbert Chasis, Robert Pitts, and Robert Berliner. He also wrote several philosophical books such as *Kamongo* —describing the lung-fish of Africa and *Man and his Gods* – with an introduction by Albert Einstein.[2] I was first introduced to Dr. Smith when I was in Medical School through his textbook, *The Kidney: Structure and Function in Health and Disease, with 2300 listed references,* published in 1951 by Oxford University Press.

Early Life

Homer Smith was born in 1895 in Denver, Colorado, the last of seven children, but spent his childhood in Cripple Creek, a small town in central Colorado. He received an A.B. degree from the University of Denver in 1917. He joined the armed forces and transferred to the Chemical Warfare Station of the American University in Washington, D.C. under Dr. E. K. Marshall to study the biological effects of nerve gases. Dr. Marshall was my Professor of Pharmacology at Hopkins in 1950. Smith and Marshall developed a lifelong friendship and Smith's first three published papers on mustard gas were published with Marshall in 1918 and 1919. After the war, Marshall arranged for Smith to undertake graduate studies at the Johns Hopkins School of Hygiene and Public Health, obtaining a Sc.D. in 1921 under William H. Howell,

---

[2] Albert Einstein, Forward to *Man and His Gods.* Homer W. Smith, Little, Brown and Company, Boston, 1952.

Professor of Physiology. The fourth published collaboration between Smith and Marshall was a long paper in the Biological Bulletin entitled *The Glomerular Development of the Vertebrate Kidney in relation to Habitat* in 1930, providing evidence that the *"protovertebrate kidney was aglomerular and that the glomerulus was evolved as an adaptation to a freshwater habitiat."* [3] These studies originated during their joint collaboration at the Marine Biological Laboratory in Maine, where both of them spent many working summers. In the Welch Library at Hopkins I found Smith's inscription in his 1937 **The Physiology of the Kidney—To E. K. Marshall from,** *Homer W. Smith, September 24, 1937.*

Further Training and Introduction to the Kidney

Working in the laboratory of Dr. Walter B. Cannon at Harvard between 1921-1923, Homer Smith devoted himself to studies of the water regulation of fish and then became chairman of the Department of Physiology at the University of Virginia College of Medicine (1925–1928). Smith continued to work in the fields of physical chemistry and cellular physiology, and it was not until 1928 that he published his first paper on a renal subject, *Note on the nitrogen excretion of camels,*

---

[3] Homer W. Smith and E.K. Marshall, Jr., The glomerular development of the vertebrate kidney in relation to habitat. Biological Bulletin, 59, 135, 1930.

published in the Journal of Biological Chemistry.[4] This was the year he was appointed Professor of Physiology and Director of the Physiological Laboratories at the New York University College of Medicine, a position he held until 1961. This short, two-and-one-half page article on the nitrogen excretion of the camel was a rather mundane correction to a previous article in the Journal by authors who had found no urea in the urine of camels, whereas Smith and his colleague Silvette found that the "camel excretes urea in amounts comparable with other herbivorous animals." This was a rather insignificant correction and gave no inkling of more important papers to follow on renal function.

Kamongo

Homer Smith's paper on the metabolism of the lung-fish in 1930 described a fish whose gills are reduced in function and can live out of water by burrowing in the mud, obtaining air in a state of hibernation or estivation. This paper provided the background for his first novel, *Kamongo,* an African word meaning lung-fish. The book published in 1932 is set in the form of a dialogue between a priest and a scientist during a slow boat trip returning from Africa. The book attained immediate popular acclaim and won many book awards for its artistry and philosophical discussion.

---

4 Homer W. Smith and H. Silvette, Note on the nitrogen excretion of camels. J. Biol. Chem., 78, 409, 1928. (This is a short article of 2 ½ pages and contradicts a previously published paper in the JBC by B.E Read who had found no urea in the urine of camels, whereas Smith and Silvette found the "camel excretes urea in amounts comparable with other herbivorous animals."

I visited Homer Smith's labs at NYU several years ago and reviewed some of his papers. *Kamongo* was enthusiastically received by the public as evidenced by the many letters Smith received. The final chapter compares life's processes to a whirlwind reflecting many of the philosophical problems which concerned Homer Smith throughout his life.

Man and His Gods

Published in 1952, *Man and His Gods*, contains a preface written by Albert Einstein. The last chapter of this book gives a graphic description of Smith's early childhood and adolescence. At the age of eleven he was given a book on chemistry. To quote Homer Smith, "In those days a knowledgeable boy could buy anything he wanted at the drugstore, from arsenic to saltpeter, and my dimes began to go into chemical experiments. Homemade gun cotton reposed casually in my trousers pocket; black powder could be compounded at any time from stock reagents on the shelves; turning water into blood by pouring it from one beaker to another, and vice versa, was kid stuff.

From Fish to Philosopher

This book was published in 1953 two years following Homer Smith's monumental *The Kidney —Structure and Function in Health and Disease,* a detailed summarization of his contributions to renal physiology. *From Fish to Philosopher* covers a variety of subjects from the evolution of the kidney to a consideration of consciousness. I found most interesting however, the chapter on the history of the development of modern renal physiology beginning in 1628 with **William Harvey's** description in *De Motu Cardis* of the "heart as a pump that keeps the blood in steady circulation around the body. "

Shortly after Harvey's death, **Lorenzo Bellini** in 1662, when he was 19 years old, described the collection duct of the kidney.

Four years later in 1666, **Marcello Malpighi,** described the glomeruli of the kidney.

Almost two centuries later in 1842 **William Bowman** using a microscope demonstrated the glomerulus draining into the tubules.

Carl Ludwig in that same year adduced the first evidence that the glomerulus acts as a minute filter carrying filtrate containing waste products into the tubule where water is reabsorbed.

In 1917 **A.R. Cushny** published the first definitive book on urine formation, *"The Secretion of the Urine."* This was followed by the work of **A.N.Richards, A.M. Walker** and **Jean Oliver** in 1933 who collected and analyzed minute quantities of fluid in Bowman's capsule and at various points in the tubule by means of micro-pipette.

The definitive demonstration of tubular secretion in 1934 was provided by **E.K. Marshall,** Smith's early mentor.

Glomerular filtration rate was reliably measured by **Homer Smith** and his group in 1938 using inulin, a soluble starch-like substance, introduced intravenously, measuring its rate of excretion.

Porter Lecture of 1939

The Porter Lecture of 1939, entitled The Evolution of the Kidney was delivered by Homer Smith at the University of Kansas Medical School, at the pre-clinical campus then located in Lawrence, Kansas. *Dr. J. L. Porter was a general practitioner from Paola, Kansas who provided for a scholarship with the balance for a lectureship.* Smith provided a brilliant analysis of how the functional architecture of the human kidney, the glomerulus and the various parts of the tubule are related to the evolution of the vertebrates, first in salt water, then fresh water and then on to dry land, all in relation to geological history beginning in the Cambrian period, 550 million years ago. Homer Smith indicates, *"the very matrix of life is water and the evolution of the kidney is essentially the story of the evolution of the regulation of water content of the body."* Or we can consider another *"one liner" from this masterful paper, " The composition of the blood is determined not by what one ingests but by what the kidneys keep."*

This figure shows the evolution of the vertebrates in relation to salt-water *(darkly-*shaded), fresh-water (lightly-shaded) and dry land in the clear area above. The time scale is at the bottom, from Cambrian period itself, 550 million years ago, when fossilized animals first began to appear.

Smith indicates that the marine invertebrates, worms, star fish, and mollusks were in osmotic equilibrium with the sea in the darkly shaded area and faced no problem of water regulation, but only the problem of the excretion of nitrogenous waste. These marine ancestors of the chordates had a pair of open ***tubules*** that connected the body cavity to the exterior, derived originally from gonaducts serving to carry the eggs and sperm out of the body to the exterior.

As the first chordates entered fresh water in the Silurian-Devonian period, the new problem was extrusion of excess water. It was necessary to devise a filtration device by bringing together arteries and these coelomic tubules to form a ***glomerulus***. *"The important point is that the renal glomerulus was evolved independently of and long after the evolution of the renal tubule."* However it was necessary to modify the tubules so that they could reabsorb the osmotically active constituents of the plasma, glucose, chloride, phosphate, etc. except for the protein which did not pass through the filtering bed of the glomerulus. *"Thus as a concomitant of the evolution of the glomerulus, there came into existence a tubule capable of reabsorbing large quantities of glucose, and similar valuable substances including sodium and chloride producing a urine hypotonic to blood."*

As reptiles with tough hides and long legs crawled onto the dry land they changed their degradation of protein nitrogen from urea to uric acid, which is almost insoluble in water. Here are the reptiles who crawled onto dry land. These reptiles secrete uric acid in the urine as a dry paste. As Smith indicates, *"This same uric acid adoption is found in birds, for the birds are but warm blooded reptiles with feathers and wings."* *My first exposure to uric acid from birds occurred when as a kid my parents took me to a* baseball game in an open stadium. My mother was wearing a broad brimmed blue hat. I noticed that on *this hat appeared a large white deposit that my father, a urologist, pointed out to me was uric acid from a bird.*

During the Mesozoic period mammals not having the propensity to degrade protein nitrogen to uric acid, continued to produce urea and developed increased circulation of the blood as an adaption for the frigidity of the environment. This resulted in increased filtration rate, entailing an increased need for conserving water by reabsorbing it from the newly emerging descending thin segment of the tubule, contributing to a hypertonic urine, the major contribution of the mammals over the last million years.

Some of the bony fish migrated back into the sea where the high pressure filtration of the glomerulus was no longer needed, shutting down the filtration function of the glomerulus, becoming an aglomerular fish.

Summary: Evolution of the Kidney

1. Marine invertebrates in the sea were in osmotic equilibrium developed **tubules** for the elimination of nitrogenous waste, 2. With entry into fresh water, **a glomerulus** developed for elimination of excess water with changes in tubular function to reabsorb glucose and electrolytes, 3. Finally there developed an ability to excrete a hypertonic urine in mammals by reabsorption of water in the **descending thin segment of the tubule.**

Homer Smith concludes *"The human kidney is far from perfect. In fact it is in many respects grossly inefficient. It begins its task by pouring some 125 ml of water into the tubules each minute, demanding for this extravagant filtration which represents a quarter of all the blood output by the heart every minute. Out of this stream of water, 99% must be reabsorbed again. This circuitous method of operation is peculiar, to say the least. At one end, the heart is working hard to pump a large quantity of water out of the body; at the other end the tubules are working equally hard to defeat the heart by keeping zero percent of this water from escaping.* Thus *the heart and kidney are literally pitched in constant battle against each other."*

The Concept of Renal Clearance

Homer Smith did not coin the expression, *clearance,* to explain a function of the kidney. In Smith's lecture on *Renal Physiology between the Two Wars,* delivered at the Mount Sinai Hospital in 1943,[5] he attributes the genesis of the term, **clearance**, to Donald D. Van Slyke, working at the Rockefeller Institute. Van Slyke was a chemist who contributed significantly to the development of nephrology, contributing 317 journal publications and five books. He worked initially at the Rockefeller Institute in New York from 1907 through 1948 and at the Brookhaven National Laboratory until 1971. His book, Quantitative Clinical Chemistry in 1931, was a collaboration with John C. Peters, Professor of Medicine at Yale University. Van Slyke's article *The Urea Clearance as a Measure of Renal Function* was published in 1936. He devised the concept of **renal clearance UV/P : The volume of plasma cleared of a substance in one minute's time,** where **U** = concentration of substance in each ml

---

[5] Homer W. Smith, The William Henry Welch Lectures 1. Renal Physiology Between Two Wars ,p. 41-57.
6. Lectures on the Didney, Porter Lectures, Series 9, University Extension Division , U. of Kansas, 1943

urine, **mg/ml** , **V** = rate of urine formation, **ml/min**, with **UV** an excretion rate in mg/min and **P** = concentration of substance in each ml plasma in **mg/ml** then **UV/P** = excretion rate/plasma concentration equals **clearance** in ml/min ie : **the volume of plasma cleared of that substance in one min.**

Homer Smith indicates, "In 1926 Van Slyke had been on his way to Baltimore to give an address to the Hopkins doctors on kidney function, and on the train his courage failed him when he thought of facing an audience again with a mathematical equation. He had learned what every lecturer must ultimately learn, that only experts can visualize and comprehend the true realities which the unreal symbols of a mathematical equation are intended to represent; the simplest equation has the fearsome power of completely dispelling the comprehension of an audience at least in the fields of medicine. As Van Slyke sat on the train seeking a solution of how to dispense with mathematics for the benefit of the medical profession , it occurred to him that all that the equation said was that in effect **some constant volume of plasma was being "cleared " of a substance in each minute of time."**

In the very next paragraph Smith indicates, *"In my opinion this word (clearance) has been more useful to renal physiology than all the equations ever written."* [6] Quoting Robert F. Pitts in his *A Biographic Memoir*, Homer William Smith realized that a precise measurement of glomerular filtration rate was central to the study of all renal functions in the

---

[6] Ibid. p. 53

intact animal, including man."[7] This he accomplished by the use of Inulin.

Current Clinical Measurement of Glomerular Filtration Rate eGFR Estimated GFR

Since glomerular filtration rate as first used by Homer Smith using IV inulin is clinically difficult to perform requiring 1. the need to start an IV, 2. achieve a constant infusion rate of Inulin, 3. take timed urine collections and blood levels. The **eGFR** or **estimated GFR** has been used in most hospitals.

One of the commonly used methods is the **CPK-Epi** equations (Chronic Kidney Disease Epidemiology Collaboration) employing the **Serum Creatinine with a negative exponent**, factoring in **age** as an exponent, **race, and sex.** This equation is complicated with negative exponents. However the chemistry lab uses a computer to do the math, recording the results without expecting a doc to learn how to use a complicated equation with negative exponents.

Clinical Studies on Renal Function as Professor of Physiology at New York University

Robert F. Pitts in his A Biographical Memoir indicates, "Homer Smith was fortunate in finding early in this phase of his career such able and devoted medical associates as Drs. Goldring, Chasis, and Shannon, and there rapidly developed a degree of intellectual exchange and stimulation between clinic and basic science. "[8]

---

[7] Robert F. Pitts. A Biographical Memoir by Robert F. Pitts, National Academy of Sciences 1967, p.53.

[8] Ibid, p. 454.

Developing a more reliable measurement of glomerular filtration rate using inulin, a non-metabolized polysaccharide containing fructose which is neither reabsorbed nor excreted by the renal tubules, proved to be an excellent choice. Para-aminohippuric acid (PAH) [9] also proved to be a similarly reliable agent to evaluate renal blood flow.[10] With these methods Smith and his clinical colleagues at NYU developed a close association between the medical clinic and the physiology department that resulted in the study of a wide variety of clinical conditions such as hypertension, renal insufficiency, and glomerulonephritis.

Homer W. Smith's Scientific Monographs Related to Renal Function and Disease

The Physiology of the Kidney, published in 1937, summarized a current analysis of kidney function including evidence for tubular secretion first described by Marshal and Crane in 1924.[11] This was the first comparable summary since the earlier publication of the British pharmacologist Arthur R. Cushny's publication, *The Secretion of the Urine* in 1917. Smith's book, *The Physiology of the Kidney, from 1937,* is an extremely readable book and Dr.

---

[9] Herbert Chasis, Jules Redish, William Goldring, Hilbert A. Ranges, and Homer W. Smith. The use of Sodium p-aminohippurate for the Functional Evaluation of the Human Kidney, Journal of Clinical Investigation, 24, 583, 1945.

[10] Homer W. Smith, William Goldring., Herbert Chasis , The measurement of the tubular mass, effective blood flow and filtration rate in normal kidney, J. Clinical Investigation 17:263: 1938

[11] Homer W. Smith, The Physiology of the Kidney, New York, Oxford University Press, 1937.

Robert Berliner indicates he was attracted to kidney research when reading this book.[12]

Homer Smith's second and really monumental treatise was entitled *The Kidney: Structure and Function in Health and Disease* was published in 1951. This book covered clinical and basic science advances in detail. I purchased a copy while in medical school and continue to refer to it. A smaller monograph, a concise, readable account of current concepts of renal function, *Principles of Renal Physiology, was* published in 1956. Homer Smith was working on a revision of this book at his death in 1962.

Summary

Homer W. Smith began his scientific career as a chemist working with Dr. E.K. Marshall during the First World War. (There followed a phase of interest in physical chemistry and cellular physiology).

He outlined the evolution of the kidney, as summarized in the Porter Lectures.

He developed a method that accurately measured glomerular filtration rate with studies using Inulin and PAH for renal blood flow. (These laboratory methods were then directed to clinical studies using these methods to evaluate renal disease, hypertension and other disorders of the kidney, bringing together the participation of many clinical departments of NYU.)

---

[12] Carl W. Gottschalk, Homer, Willam Smith: A Remembrance, J. AM. Soc. Nephrol, 5, 1985, 1995.

Homer Smith summarized his findings in the monumental book: *The Kidney: Structure and Function in Health and Disease in 1951.*

5. Philosophical considerations of man's place in the universe occupied his interests as well. The publication of *Kamongo in 1932* brought together his findings on the lung- fish as well a discussion of man's place in the universe and human consciousness. (Other books along these lines include *From Fish to Philosopher* and *Man and His Gods.)*

6. Other subjects considered were the concept of renal clearance, eGFG, and review of the history of the development of renal physiology beginning in 1628 with William Harvey's description of the heart as a pump.

7. In 1967 Robert F. Pitts, a student of Homer Smith, wrote a Bibliographical Memoir which indicates that "The characteristics which set Homer W. Smith apart from his peers were the rapidity with which he could grasp an involved concept, examine its several facets, marshal a variety of arguments in favor of and against it, and quickly return it to its proponents, simplified and stripped of inconsequential trappings."

Chapter Seven

John C. Hemmeter, MD; PHD; Sc.D.;
LL.D., 1863-1931
Professor of Physiology and Clinical
Professor of Medicine and Regent at
University of Maryland

This essay includes a brief evaluation of John C
Hemmeter's work, interests, and multiple contacts
among leaders of medicine.

My first acquaintance with John C. Hemmeter
occurred when I was trying to write a paper on
Theodor Billroth and stumbled across a paper by
Hemmeter read before the Johns Hopkins Hospital
Historical Club and published in the Johns
Hopkins Bulletin, December 1900. This paper
occupying 46 pages in Hemmeter's magnificent
book, *Masterminds in Medicine,* was published in
1927 by the New York Medical Live Press.

After I studied Hemmeter's article on Theodor BillrothI was inspired to leanr more about John C. Hemmeter, his work and savor his rich associations with leaders of medicine of his day.

John C Hemmeter was born in Baltimore, Maryland. His parents were from Germany and he spent several years of his early education in Weisbaden Germany. He attended high school at Baltimore City College and medical school at the University of Maryland graduating in 1884. He became interested in gastroenterology and ecame Professor of Physiology at the University of Maryland. He received a PhD in Physiology from Johns Hopkins in 1890 and a LLD from St. Johns College in 1905. He was a contemporary and friendly with many of the Hopkins early physicians such as Welch, Halsted, Mall, Osler, and Abel as well as Garrison. He spent time in Woods Hole in Massachusetts also.

His early home was at 1739 Linden Avenue in downtown Baltimore, later moving to a house at 739 University Parkway, near where I currently live in Roland Park.

He was interested in music and wrote a Cantata, "Hygeia" for male chorus and grand orchestra widely produced I the larger Eastern cities. He was the author of numerous compositions for voices, piano and instruments. According to Henry Elliot Shepherd, AM and LLD who wrote "the Musical Contributions of a Physiologist," quoting Asger Hammeter, "it was very much to be regretted that Hemmeter had devoted himself to medicine at all because music had lost a most promising scholar and composer, who might have originitated compositions of enduring value."

Hemmeter wrote many articles published in the Johns Hopkins Bulletin such as "Lavoisier and the History of the Physiology of Respiration and Metabolism. Contemporary views of Life Processes." He also authored, "Albrecht von Haller: Scientific Literary and Poetical Activity" in March 1906 edition. Additional articles were published in the Philadelphia Medical Journal of 5/1/1901 on the German Clinics of Today and in the John Hopkins Bulletin of May 1905, History of Circulation of the Blood, Contributions of the Italian Anatomist. In the Johns Hopkins Bulletin of 1896 on page 79, opposite and article by Dr. Osler is an article by Hemmeter on "Intubation of the Duodenum."

However most interesting are the letters that Hemmeter wrote or received from a variety of other well known physicians such as William H. Welch, Halsted, John Abel, and MacCullum:

January 19, 1929 "Dr. William H. Welch, Brow Shipley and Co. London England"
Dear Dr. Welch

When Dr. McCallum told us about your experiences abroad and the interesting but very responsible duty of selecting books with the fund that you had been authorized to spend on this, it occurred to me that I had better consult you concerning a number of things about the coming meeting of the American Section of the International society for the History of Medicine." Going on for 2 pages and concluding with:

"The canon of human proportions from Polyclitus, a contemporary of Phidias, to Leonardo da Vinci and Albrecht Durer has occupied most of the studies this winter, but I am also thinking out the plan to a lexicon of medical history in three categories: (1) first, chronologically, (2) second a biographically organized section, and (3) thirdly subject-matter, each as condensed and abstract in form as possible. I felt the need of a work like this when I was engaged with my Master Minds of Medicine

Signed With Best Regards, Yours faithfully
John C. Hemmeter

November 24th, 1918
Dear Dr. Halsted:

It appears he has an intrathoracic thyroid which is at the level of the 4rt rib. There are no chemotoxic symptoms such as hyperthyroidism. The chief signs are mechanical consequences, due to compression. I would like to speak with MCCallum after I see you next Thursday at 12:20 pm.

Signed with Best Regards, Yours Faithfully
John C. Hemmeter

Nov. 10th, 1920
Dear Dr. Welch:
After discussion with Dr. Edward C. Streeter of Boston, Col Fielding H. Garrison of the Surgeon-General's library and Dr. Howard A Kelly of Baltimore, I have conveived a plan of organizing a new section in the American Medical Association to be called "the section of medical history." It would

be a federation of physicians interested in medical history, with the advantage that no additional dues beyond those paid to the AMA would be necessary meeting annually and affording opportunity to stimulate the preparation of good papers for the occasion, etc. Hoping you are well, with best regards I am faithfully yours
John C Hemmeter

Aug 30th, 1929
Dear Dr. MacCallum:

Thanks for the invitation to the dedication o the Welch Medical Library and the Department of the History of Medcine. Mrs. Hemmeter and myself accept with pleasure. Owing to the presence of of Sudhoff I have suggested to Dr. Goodnow and to Dr. Welch tha thte Ambassador of Germany be sent an invitation. Etc.

With best Regards, Cordially Yours,
John C. Hemmeter

A very brief note from William Osler dated 1916

Dear John:
How is it with you? All right I hope. Did you go north? Let me know if you do that. I may send introductions. With Best wishes
W. Osler

Finally a letter to Dr. John Abel, dated Dec. 27, 1917

Dear Dr. Abel:
A membership in the Society for Pharmacology and Experimental Therapeutics would be a help toward keeping me up to date on the newer way of

understanding the effect of chemical substances on the cells, etc. Compliments for the Season from yours faithfully,
John C. Hemmeter

Such are some of the letter exchanges to a variety of friends and colleagues of Hemmeter: Dr.s Welch, Halsted, MacCallum, and Abel- all Hopkins Professors as well as a brief letter from William Osler.

Master Minds of Medicine

Hemmeter's 771 page book, Master Minds in Medicine which was published in 1927 with an introduction by Karl Sudoff, MD was dedicated to Charles Horace Mayo and William James Mayo of Rochester Minnesota. It states, "because you have been leaders of great constructive ideas, brilliant contributions to medical and Surgical Science and Are inspiring Teachers, and above all great lovers of mankind, this volume is dedicated to you by the Author as a contemporaneous token of the loyalty that History will sustain and future generations will approve."

The preface begins," the reciprocal relationship between master minds which the human race has produced and Society at large has not received the concentrated study witch this great problem deserves, etc. on 13 pages

Then there is an introduction of 5 pages beginning y Carl Sudhoff , "My friend Hemmeter, requests me to contribute a few remarks as an introduction to his Master Minds of Medicine. I am delighted to accede him this request, etc.

Then thirty three chapters beginning with Methodology in Medical Historiography for 33 pages beginning with "medical historiography can be found upon a basic stock of facts and truths, in which the manifold and different sources are clearly concordant and from which any possibility of fraud or counterfeit can be excluded and therefore the synthetic deductions be accepted as indubitable, etc.

Then 41 pages on (1) Medical Versus General History is followed by a 37 pages on (2) Ideas as Factors in Medical History followed by 19 pages on (3) the Role and Function of Great scientists in Medical History followed by (4) the Criteria of what constitutes a great medical discovery or invention, and then (5) Statistics in histiiography followed by (6) Medicine in the 20th Century and finally to the chapter which drew me initially to the book: (7) Theodor Billroth, Musical and Surgical Philosopher for 46 pages.

The chapters on the history of the circulation of the blood, Rudolf Virchow, Albrecht Von Haller and then we are less than half way through this large tome!

Hemmetter's Germanic systematic comprehensiveness is remarkable! His work flows logically from section to section. It is clearly a monumental undertaking and a testament to the wide scope of his knowledge of the history of medicine

Summary

John C. Hemmeter MD PHD, SC.D, LL.D was a Professor of Physiology and Gastroenterologist at the University of Maryland in Baltimore City.

He was a contemporary and friendly with many of the Hopkins early physicians and medical elite such as Drs. Welch, Halsted, Mall, Osler, and Abel, as well as others including Dr. Garrison.

He was interested in music and wrote a cantata, "Hygeia" for male chorus and orchestra displaying a great well roundedness in science and music

He published many articles such as Lavoisier and the History of Physiology of Respiration" ad "Albrecht von Haller: Scientific Literary, and Poetical Activity" published in the Johns Hopkins Bulletin.

He wrote many letters to Hopkins physicians such as Drs. Welch, Halsted, Abel, MacCullum and received a note from Dr. William Osler.

His book, "Master Minds in Medicine" was published in 1927 with introduction by Karl Sudhoff. It consisted of 771 pages dedicated to the Mayo Brothers of Rochester, Minnesota including introductory chapters on Methodology in Medical Historiography, Sources of Medical History, Great Men in Medical History with a most delightful chapter on Dr. Theodor Billroth, History of Recognition in Gastric Ulcer, Science and the Art in Medicine among many others

Chapter Eight

William A. Marburg's Contribution to Sir William Osler's Love for Books and Libraries

(with Christine Rugere)

William Osler was well known as a lover of books and promoter of Libraries and this paper documents the role of William A. Marburg, a business man and Vice President of the Johns Hopkins Hospital for many years, in obtaining collections for the Johns Hopkins Medical School Library in the early 20th Century.

Osler's interests in Books and Libraries

Medicine and books were a lifelong obsession for William Osler. In *Books and Men* an address he gave in 1901 at the opening of the new building of the Boston Medical Library Osler indicates, *"It is hard for me to speak of the value of libraries in terms which would not seem exaggerated. Books have been my delight these thirty years, and from them I have received incalculable benefits. To study the phenomena of disease without books is to sail an uncharted sea, while to study books without patients is not to go to sea at all."[1]* A visit to the medical library in every city he visited was a routine. He was a great collector of medical books, especially first editions. He purchased a first edition of Sir Thomas Browne's *Religio Medici* from 1643 in August 1899 and at Osler's death in 1919 had accumulated all 69 editions that are neatly displayed in a case to the right of the niche containing his plaques and ashes at the McGill Osler library.

Quoting from the prologue of *Bibliotheca Osleriana*, *"In Harvey Cushing's 'Life of Sir William Osler some forty libraries are listed by name in the index. Perhaps half a dozen of these are casual references, but many point to long and cherished associations, and a few, such as the entries for the Boston Medical Library, the College of Physicians Library in Philadelphia, or the Medical and Chirurgical Faculty of Maryland Library , indicate special personal commitments. All this leaves out of account the libraries of McGill, the University of Pennsylvania, Johns Hopkins and Oxford. Nor is it certain that even the longer list is complete. The private libraries of Johnson and Bovell (boyhood mentors in Canada) helped to satisfy Osler's curiosity and to form his taste at early stages in his career, and thereafter, wherever he went – Montreal, Philadelphia, Baltimore, Oxford – he not only sought out and used the libraries, he became in almost every case an active and generous friend."* [2]

---

[1] Aequanimitas, Xll, Books and Men, p.220.

[2] Bibliotheca Osleriana, Prologue, p. lX

According to Cushing in his biography of Osler, *"His interest in libraries was cumulative and a contact once made was never subsequently lost. The libraries at McGill, that of the Surgeon-General in Washington, of the College of Physicians in Philadelphia, of the Johns Hopkins Hospital and many others which he perhaps knew less intimately, all continued to profit by his unflagging support-moral and often financial.*[3] He was often fond of giving rare books to libraries and Hopkins has a copy of his first edition of William Harvey's *De Motu Cordis.*

On coming to Baltimore Osler established relationship with the fledgling Medical and Chirurgical Faculty of Maryland and became a member of the Library committee in 1892. He was instrumental in increasing the size of the library form a few thousand books in 1892 to over 14,000 volumes in 1905 when he left Baltimore.[4] He was instrumental in the moving of the library to an elegant building at 1211 Cathedral street, increasing its endowment and employing a full time librarian. The main meeting hall is currently called Osler Hall containing a beautiful picture of Osler.

Osler was familiar with auctions of books and libraries and in 1906 wanting to augment the fledgling library of the Johns Hopkins Hospital noted an auction at the London bookseller, Sawyer, containing sixteenth through eighteenth century books collected by the physicians connected with the Warrington Dispensary in England. Osler

---

[3] Cushing, Harvey, The Life of Sir William Osler, 1 94 0, p. 344.

[4] Noyes, Marcia C. Osler's Influence on the Library of the Medical Chirurgical Faculty of the State of Maryland. Johns Hopkins Hospital Bulletin , p.212

suggested that William A. Marburg buy it for the Johns Hopkins Medical School. Who was William A. Marburg and why did Osler pick him to finance this collection of these 1200 rare books?

William A. Marburg

William A. Marburg (1849-1930) was born in Baltimore. His grandfather was a successful merchant in Germany and his father born in Germany in 1814 came to Baltimore at age 16 in 1830. William was a student at the Knapp's Institute in Baltimore and with this two brothers, Charles L and Louis H. joined in the business to manufacture smoking tobacco. A younger brother, Theodore joined in this enterprise and in 1923 founded the Johns Hopkins Faculty Club at Homewood in Baltimore. Interestingly the other German family of note in Baltimore at this time was the Mencken family which also was in the tobacco manufacturing business. Henry L.Mencken (1880–1946) who also attended the Knapp Institute [5]was strongly encouraged to join his father in the

---

[5] Teachout, Terry, The Skeptic, A Life of H. L. Mencken, 2002, p. 32. "Harry (H.L. Mencken) was poor at sports, but he could read by the age of three and write by the time he was five. In September 1866, he entered F. Knapp's Institute, a private school across from City Hall in downtown Baltimore, some two miles from Hollins Street. (He rode there by streetcar every day). ...Too clumsy to shine on the playground, he concentrated on his studies, and his first term report card, dated December 24, 1886, shows the results: :Deportment: Excellent. Industry: Praiseworthy. Advancement: Very satisfactory. Cleanliness: Very neat. The ponderous teaching methods of Friedrich Knapp and his staff appear to have had little impact on Harry, who later claimed (in typical Menckenese) that "the professor and his goons certainly never taught me to speak German, or even to read it with any ease."

tobacco business but as a teenager H.L. Mencken would have none of it and found his way as a junior reporter on a local newspaper rising to become the sage of Baltimore. William A Marburg and his brothers eventually sold out to the American Tobacco Company in 1891 with William elected as vice president. In addition to serving as director of several business and the National Union Bank in Baltimore, William A Marburg served as vice president and trustee of the Johns Hopkins Hospital for many years. His large portrait hangs in the foyer of the Hospital along with Johns Hopkins and John Shaw Billings among others. Following taking up Osler on bankrolling the Warrington Dispensary collection of books William A. had supported the building of the Marburg Pavilion, for a total of $ 5,025,000 an area for private patients that stands today with its iron railed porches.

The Warrington Dispensary Library

William Osler in an article entitled *On the Library of a Medical School* from April 1907, on the occasion of the presentation of the Marburg collection of books to the Johns Hopkins medical School in the Bulletin of The Johns Hopkins Hospital, describes the collection of books he had recommended that William A. Marburg purchased:

"One day last spring a London Bookseller called and said he had a library of seventeenth and eighteenth century medical books for sale, which had been gathered by the physicians connected with the Warrington Dispensary. Looking over the catalogue I was at once that it was a collection of value, and knowing that it would supplement very nicely the specially libraries which have gradually grown up in connection with the

Johns Hopkins Medical School, I wrote to Mr. W.A. Marburg and he authorized me to purchase it and to have it put in good order, and this has been done, and to complete this generous gift, Mr. Marburg has furnished bookcases as well."

Osler describes Warrington as "This old town on the banks of the Mersey, partly in Chester, partly in Lancashire, had in the middle and latter part of the eighteenth century a notable group of scientific and professional men. " Rather than describe the actual books or authors, Osler is more interested in this "notable group of scientific and professional men" who had lived at Warrington. First there was the Aiken family, through the Rev. John Aiken "that the Warrington Academy became so famous." Osler emphasizes however it was Joseph Priestly "who was tutored in classics and polite literature at the academy for six years, from 1761." Osler indicates that Thomas Percival was born in Warrington and practiced there before going to Manchester. Osler conclude, " Altogether, the collection has an affiliation with a remarkable group of men, and its value is not a little enhanced to know that it has been used by such men as Priestly, John Aiken and Thomas Percival." [6]

At the end of article on the Warrington collection on the occasion of the presentation of the Marburg collection, Osler indicates, *"In practical illustration of my remarks I beg to present to the Marburg collection an original edition of the 'De Motu Cordis' 1626, perhaps the greatest single contribution to medicine ever*

---

[6] Osler, William, On the Library of a Medical School, Bulletin of the Johns Hopkins Hospital, Vol XVIII, #193, April 1907, p. 109-110. Remarks made on the occasion of the presentation of the Marburg collection of books to the Johns Hopkins Medical School, Jan2, 1907.

made, and which did as much for physiology as the 'Fabrica' of Vesalius did for anatomy."

Accompanying this article by Olser in the Bulletin of the Johns Hopkins Hospital of 1907 on this occasion, is an article by M. L. Raney, Assistant Librarian of the Johns Hopkins University, describing the collection. Half of the collection of 1000 books was published before 1750, thirty three titles in the sixteenth century of which Vigo's Opera ...in chyrurgia (Works on Surgery) is the oldest form 1531. There is a Burton's Anatomy of Melancholy of which Raney states, "Ours is a beautiful copy, though the eight edition of 1676, the edition princeps (original edition) belonging to the year 1621.

R. Guest-Gornall has written a description of the Warrington Dispensary Library.[7] He describes one particular manuscript lectures of John Rutherford , maternal grandfather of Sir Walter Scott. Guest-Gornall indicates, *"Osler must have prized this unpretentious volume, as, though stamped with the Dispensary mark, he never let it reach Baltimore but kept it to himself so that it passed eventually to the Osler Library at McGill University."* [8] There it rests to this day, having missed the trip to the Hopkins Library as part of the Warrington Collection. Osler indicates that he personally paid for this volume and considered it specially because of it having been said to have been used by Hermann Boerhaave. Perhaps we can forgive Osler for pirating away this particular volume to his alma

---

[7] Guest-Gornall, R., Medical History, v. 11(3); July 1967, p285-300.

[8] Ibid. p. 293.

martyr, McGill, with his gift to Hopkins on the dedication of the Marburg Collection of the *Motu Cordis*.

Jonathan Hutchinson's Collection

Jonathan Hutchinson (1828–1913) was an English surgeon with a wide ranging interest and observer in multiple fields. He was president of the Royal College of Surgeons in 1888. "His interests and clinical activities knew no bounds and reached far beyond what is generally considered the province of surgeons."[9] He had a penchant for the rare and unique. As William Osler, a great admirer of Hutchinson indicated, "When anything turns up which is an anomaly or peculiar, anything upon which the textbooks are silent and the systems and cyclopaedias are dumb, I tell my students to turn to the volumes of Mr. Hutchinson's Archives of Surgery as , if it is not mentioned in them, it surely is something very much out of the common."[10] His field of observation and interest included neurological, dermatological including syphilis, ophthalmalogical and genetic studies. He had available an artist illustrator, Edwin Burgess, who recorded unusual and interesting findings that that were published in his Archives of Surgery from 1890 through 1900. " As pathologist, surgeon, syphilographer, neurologist, dermatologist, ophthalmologist, allergist and collector of all that is

---

[9] McKusick, Victor A., The Clinical Observations of Jonathan Hutchinson, American Journal of Syphilis, Gonorrhea, and Venereal Diseses. Vol36, #2 p. 101-102.

[10] Osler, W. The importance of post-graduate study, Lancet, 1900, 2 p.73.

curious and unusual in medicine, he made in each field significant major contributions together with numerous lesser ones." [11]

William Osler / William A Marburg Combination Again to the Rescue of a Clinical Collection

Jonathan Hutchinson's clinical career is provided by his "Clinical Museum containing an extensive collection of illustration, some photographic, but mostly water colors, by illustrators Edwin Burgess, Mabel Green and others. After Hutchinson's death in 1913, the collection of clinical illustrations and case reports was acquired by the Johns Hopkins Medical School through the agency of Sir William Osler and the financial generosity of Mr. W. A., Marburg of Baltimore. The collection arrived in Baltimore in 1915 in eight large crates (with British war bond posters covering the material). In that year Osler published a small note in the Johns Hopkins Hospital Bulletin describing the collection:[12]

(It) illustrates the whole of medicine and surgery…The drawings are classified: one group comprising more than 5,000 are in large paper envelopes, the other an even larger number, in large cardboard portfolios. while they illustrate particularly the life work of the collector in syphilis and skin diseases, there is scarcely a department

---

[11] Mckusick, Victor, A. The Clinical Observations of Jonathan Hutchinson. American Journal of Syphilis, Gonorrhea and Venereal Disease. Vol 36, #2 p. 102.

[12] Mckusik, Victor, A. The Gordon Wilson Lecture: the Clinical Legacy of Jonathan Hutchinson (1818-1931): Syndromotology and Dysmorphology Meets Genomics, Trahsactions of the American Clinical and Climatological Association. 116, 2005, p. 1 and 2.

of medicine that has not one or two portfolios devoted to it."[13]

Osler had had many meetings with Hutchinson and admired his work and clinical acumen as documented by the many references in Cushing's biography of Osler, such as at the meeting of the International Association of Medical Museums where in 1913 where "Osler, prefacing his remarks by a warm tribute to the late Sir Jonathan Hutchinson, *"at whose wonderfully popular museum at Haslemere the results produced by the classification of well-chosen material along any line might be seen. "[14]*

Victor A. Mckusick's Use of the Hutchinson Collection at Johns Hopkins

Dr. Mukusick indicates that *"In the academic year 1950-51, while a senior assistant resident on the Osler Medical Service, I devoted all of the spare time I could to a review both of the Hutchinson collection (then reposing still in the eight crates in the Welch Medical Library) and of Hutchinson's numerous publications. On the basis of these, I produced a 25 page article entitled, "The clinical observations of Jonathan Hutchinson illustrated with items from the Clinical Museum. [15]*

---

[13] Osler, William, The iconography of Jonathan Hutchinson, Bulletin Johns Hopkins Hospital. 26 1915, p. 82.

[14] Cushing, Harvey, The Life of Sir William Osler, 1940, p. 1055, but also see p 980, 1164, 919, "the last of the polymaths, the man at home in all spheres of medical science."

[15] McKusick, Victor A., The Gordon Wilson Lecture: The Clinical Legacy of Jonathan Hutchinson: Syndromology and Dysmorphology Meet Genomics, Trans Am Clin Climatol Assoc 116, 2005, , p. 2.

I remember as a medical student at Hopkins in 1951 hearing Mckusick speak on Johnathan Hutchison at the Welch Library and for the first time hearing and seeing pictures of *Mortimer's Malady* (Hutchinson was fond of naming a newly discovered condition after the name of the patient he first saw the condition)–a cutaneous form of Boeck's sarcoid and *Hutchinson's teeth*- pointed incisors of congenital syphilis.

McKusick indicated his interested in Jonathan Hutchinson in June 1947 when on the final month of his Osler internship, *"I was introduced to the polyps-and Spot syndrome by a teen aged patient, Harold Parker. The patient had the characteristic pigmentary changes and during the first decade of life had chronic anemia with jejuna polyps discovered."* [16] In 1896 Hutchinson had reported identical twins with cutaneous features of the polyps-and –spot syndrome.[17] Harold Jegers then in Boston had seen five such cases and McKusick and Jegers reported these cases in the New England Journal of Medicine in 1949[18]. The syndrome subsequently has been called the Peutz-Jegers syndrome. McKusick's recognition of Hutchinson's description of the skin lesions of this hereditary condition may have been the stimulus for his future career in hereditary disease.

---

[16] Ibid. p3.

[17] Hutchinson J. Records of demonstrations at the Clinical Museum. Pigmentation of the lips and mouth. Arch. Surg. 7, 1896, p286-294.

[18] Jegers H, McKusick VA, Katz KH, Generalized intestinal polyposis and melanin spots of the oral mucosa, lips and digits. New Eng. J. Med 241, 1949, p. 993-1005.

A Collection that Got Away from William Osler and William A. Marburg

Not all of the library auction snooping that Osler engaged in proved as successful as the Warrington Collection or the Jonathan Hutchinson collections that made their way to Hopkins. In the Bibliotheca Historica, a description of Osler's catalogue of books on the history of medicine collected, arranged an annotated by Sir William Osler under item #6350.[19]

*"Catalogue of the.collection of early Medical Works... also.. Books and Tracts on pestilence... the property of John Frank Payne...which will be sold by auction...July, 1911...la.8 (Lond. 1911). I was anxious that the library should be kept together, and my friend, M. W.A. Marburg, of Baltimore, very kindly commissioned me to buy it for the Johns Hopkins Medical School, for which a few years ago he bought a valuable collection of old books. The executors had placed a reserve price of L 2,700 but on the morning of the sale I received an intimation that it would be reduced to L 2,500. The collection was to be offered first en block. With Dr. Henry Barton Jacobs and Dr. George Dock, I went to Sotheby's at one o'clock on July 12th. **A more rapid sale I never saw!** The bidding began at L 2,000, and within a minute it was knocked down to an unknown bidder at L 2,300, a figure beyond that which Mr. Marburg had mentioned, but Dr. Jacobs and I were prepared to go to the 'reserve price, **had we had a chance.** The library went to the Wellcome Historical Museum, London.*

---

[19] Bibliotheca Osleriana, Osler, William, McGill-Queen's University Press , p.552. #6350.

In the Preface to the Biblioteca Osleriana, Osler concludes, "There were many good items in the collection, and I am glad for the sake of Dr. Payne's memory that it has been kept together and well housed in the Wellcome Historical Museum."[20]

Summary

Sir William Osler was devoted to the collecting of books from his youth. The thrill and allure of old books were as challenging as a clinical problem in diagnosis or treatment. Recall his feelings with regard to books in the article *Books and Men*, "*Books have been my delight these thirty years, and from them I have received incalculable benefits. To study the phenomena of disease without books is to sail an uncharted sea, while to study books without patients is not to go to sea at all.*"

This paper has documented the roll of William A. Marburg, a Baltimore tobacco manufacturer in bank rolling Osler recommendations in purchasing the Warrington Dispensary Library in 1906, a collection approaching a thousand books from the 16th through the 18th century , half before 1750 and 33 titles from the sixteenth century. The second joint cooperation between Osler and Marburg was the Jonathan Hutchinson's Collection in 1915, comprising over 5000 items on a variety of subjects Hutchinson had collected relating to dermatological, neurological, genetic and unusual finding in syphilis and other subjects. Dr. Victor Mckusick reviewed this material and may have been a stimulus for his subsequent interest in hereditable disease.

---

[20] Ibid Preface, p. 5.

Finally the Osler–Marburg combination missed out on one auction of the Payne collection because of a *"rapid sale"* at auction yet Osler was *"glad for the sake of Dr. Payne that his collection has been kept together and well housed at the Wellcome Historical Museum."*

Chapter Nine

Osler's mention of Basham's Mixture
William Osler's Mention of Basham's
Mixture in the Treatment of Bright's
Disease
Who was Basham and what was his
Mixture?

Basham's mixture given in plenty of water well be found beneficial. (Osler, William, Principles and Practices of Medicine, final sentence of paragraph on Treatment of Chronic Parenchymatous Nephritis, p. 704, 1892.

The full quotation concerning Basham's mixture under Treatment of Chronic Parenchymatous Nephritis (large white kidney with marked dropsy, abundant albumin, ie: nephrotic syndrome) is quoted from Osler's text from 1892:

Essentially the same treatment should be carried out as in acute Bright's Disease. Milk or buttermilk should constitute for a time the chief article of food. Later more food may be allowed oysters, fresh vegetables, and fruits.

The dropsy should be treated by the hot baths, and a <u>salt free diet</u>. Iron preparations should be given when there is marked anaemia. It is to be remembered that the pallor of the face may not be a good index of the blood condition. The acetate of potash, digitalis and diuretin (theobrominae) *are useful in increasing the flow of urine.* **Basham's mixture given in plenty of water will be found beneficial.**

Who was Basham and what was the nature of his mixture? This paper will place William Basham in the line of the history of nephrology following Richard Bright's salient paper in 1827, *Reports of Medical Case.* He employed the emerging use of the microscope and the concept of cellular pathology resulting in changes in therapy including the rational for the use of Basham's mixture.

William Richard Basham (1804 – 1877) was born in Diss, a town of 6,700 in north eastern England in Norfolk. It lies in the valley of the River Waveney , around a lake or *mere,* the town taking its name from the Saxon for lake. It is an ancient town, including an early 14th century parish church. It was not until 1831 when he was 27 years old that he enrolled as a student at Westminster Hospital and graduated as a physician a year later from Edinburgh, where Richard Bright and most all English physicians at that time received there medical degrees. Like Bright who took a tour of the continent, Vienna and Hungry before starting practice, Basham made a voyage in the East India Company's ship *Hythe* to China and was wounded in a skirmish. On his return to England it was not until 1843 that he secured the appointment of physician to the Westminter Hospital. Basham became best known for his work on renal diseases., publishing *On Dropsy, and its connection with Diseases of the Kidneys, Heart, Lungs, and Liver* in the year 1858, the year of Richard Bright's death. To quote from Basham's dedication to Richard Bright in this volume:

To Richard Bright, M.D., F.R.S., etc., etc.
Dear Sir: The pathology of the disease which you were the first to describe, and which is inseparable associated with you name, has engaged the attention of many inquirers. The disease has been examined from various points of view, and much as been done to elucidate its causes, its complications ,and its progress. The subject however, is not exhausted; and in the following pages I have endeavoured to remove some of the obscurity which still surrounds several points connected with this disease.

It is with sincere and grateful respect that I dedicate these pages to you, animated with the hope that they may assist to place on a true basis the pathology of the disease which bears your name, and contribute to our knowledge of the foretokens of these diseases of the kidney.

I am,
Dear Sir,
Very faithfully yours,

W.R. Basham
17, Chester Street Grosvenor Place
August 21st, 1858

Bright's recognition of a clinical entity of dropsy and coagulable urine related to renal pathology at autopsy received little recognition initially by his colleagues in London but rather recognition came from Scotland by Robert Christison in his *On Granular Degeneration of the Kidnies,* in 1839. Christison set the tone of doubt over the significance of the finding, stating that Bright's discoveries *"were received at first with coldness by his brethren. It was said that such cases as he described had been seen only in Guy's Hospital, and in the scum alone of the London population."* [1] In Ireland, Jonathan Osborne (1834) and in France, Pierre Rayer (1839) equally recognized Richard Bright's contributions. But in England it was not until 1858 that William Basham became an equally enthusiastic supporter, *"It is little beyond thirty years since our distinguished countryman, Dr. Bright, laid the foundation by his invaluable and original observations, for a more correct knowledge of these forms of dropsy."*[2]

Like Richard Bright, an accomplished water-color painter, Basham was an excellent draughtsman and many of his illustrations drawn from microscopic appearance of casts in tubules and epithelial lining cells appear in his works. In addition to *On Dropsy,* Basham published a compact volume *Renal Diseases, A Clinical Guide* in 1870, a handbook for the clinician and student. It is in his Croonian Lectures of 1864 on the *Significance of Dropsy* that Basham summaries his approach to dropsy and renal diseases and promulgates his formulation of an iron preparation, thereafter designated as Basham's mixture.

---

[1] Christison, Robert, On granular Degeneration of th Kidnies, and its Connection with Dropsy, Inflammations, and other Diseases, 1839, p.

[2] Basham,William, Croonian lectures, Lecture 1, 1865, p. 6.

The theme of the first lecture was, "whether our modern methods of investigation *by microscope research are calculated to obtain for us a wider significance for dropsical diseases than has hitherto been accorded to them.*" Richard Bright's 1827 *Reports of Medical Cases selected with a View of Illustrating the Symptoms and Cure of Diseases by a Reference to Morbid Anatomy,* was based on gross pathological findings and clinical observation of dropsy and coagulable urine. The unavailability of achromatic microscopic lenses made examination of urine and sections of the kidney not possible.[3] Basham indicated in the first Croonian lecture, "*Bright, however, lived to witness the application of more minute methods of research, and he appreciated highly the results which the microscope was yielding to those who followed in the path he had opened.*"[4] Basham had the advantage of being able to use the microscope to study urine and tissue sections, now that achromatic lenses were available and an adequate microtome was available to cut appropriately thin sections of tissue. These factors plus the concept of cellular pathology, advocated by Vichow and others added a new dimension to evaluating underlying disease processes. Basham was to take advantage of these two advances, use of the

---

[3] The paper by Cameron J.S, Becker E.L., Richard Bright and observations in renal history, *Guy's Hospital Reports* 1964, 113, 159-71. does quote a letter from Bright indicating that he and his student, Mr. J. Toynbee have been carrying our microscopic observations on the changes in structure of the kidney with the progression of disease. However Bright's name does not appear on the paper eventually published by Toynbee, On the intimate studies of the human kidney, and on the changes which its several components parts undergo in "Bright disease, *Transactions of the Royal Medical Chirurgical Society of London, 1846, 29, 303-24.*

[4] Basham, William, R, Croonian lectures, Lecture 1, 1864, p. 6

microscope and importance of cellular patholgy, to look at Bright's Disease in a new way in his text, *On Dropsy,* and summarized in his Croonian lectures.

In this first chapter from the Croonian lectures of 1864, Basham discusses the etiology of dropsy as not being a disease in itself as had previously been considered. He considers three causes of dropsical effusion: 1. "a poor, watery, exhausted blood, a blood deficient in red corpusles, but abounding in white colourless cells (white cells), 2. Presence in the blood of "excrementitious or other noxious material" as might occur in scarlet-fever or with accumulation of urea with impaired renal function, 3. Impediments to the free passage of blood through one or other of the great organ, heart lungs or liver. These naïve causes of dropsy with out demonstrative proof are Basham's alternative to considering dropsy as a disease in itself, as had been considered in the past.

Compare this concept of Dropsy to that of John Elliotson as appears in his 1843 edition of *The Principles and Practice of Medicine* (antedating William Osler's textbook of the same name by forty nine years):[5]

Definition of Dropsy: The next class of affections that we have to consider, belong entirely to serous membranes, and the intestines of the serous cellular tissue. In these cases fluid is secreted in such excess that the ordinary processes of absorption are inadequate for its removal and as the serous cavities of the body are shut sacs, the fluid does not escape, as it does from mucous

---

[5]   Elliotson, John, The Principles and Practice of Medicine, 1843, p. 146.

membranes, so that instead of a discharge or flux, dropsy is the result.

Basham's considers dropsy as more then a condition of the serous membranes but the concept of renal sodium retention as a cause of dropsy would require a more physiological approach to be developed in the future.

Basham then does on to his main thesis that "it is to the very general employment of the microscope in the examination of the excretions during life, as well as of the structure of the organs and tissues after death that we must trace the greater part of the progress that is now being made in the pathology and treatment of these diseases."[6] He credits Virchow and Henle at the University of Berlin stating "that we are chiefly indebted for the extension of the physiology of the cells to the interpretation of the phenomena of disease." While the English lagged behind the European countries in cellular pathology he credits the English school of Mr. Bowman, and Drs. William Addison and Lionel Beale for making advances in this field as well.[7]

Basham gives credit to Dr. Bright who laid the foundations by post-mortem investigation of the significance of the kidneys in the diseases leading to dropsy. However these gross methods of

---

[6] Ibid, p.6.

[7] Lionel Smith Beale(1828-1906) was instrumental in furthering the use of the microscope with his publications *The Microscope in Medicine and How to work with the Microscope*. William Osler used as a student and retained a copy of the later in his library and wrote an obituary in Lancet, 1906, 1, 1004.

pathology were recognized to have their limits as the microscope provided clues to further information. He continues in this regard, "We find that in every direction in which microscopic research has been hitherto made, evidence has been obtained of alteration in the character of the cellular elements – often times proportioned to, and characteristic of special morbid processes. He recognized that "after Mr. Bowman's description of the basement membrane" or what he calls the germinal membrane is responsible for the succession of single layer of cells forming the renal tubule. "In the early stage of renal disturbance accompanied by albuminous urine and dropsy, the epithelial gland structure of the renal tubes exhibits the simplest and earliest departure from the healthy or physiological type." Plates with drawings by Basham of these changes which are delicate and meticulously drawn accompany the lectures.

Basham puts it succinctly, "The microscope, therefore, as an instrument of investigation should be to the diseases of the kidney, what the stethoscope is to the diseases of the lungs."[8] He discusses changes in the epithelial cells of the tubules with the development of granular and fatty changes and as the disease progresses finally sloughing off in the form of casts that can be examined under the microscope. This would allow

---

[8] Basham, W.R., On Dropsy, and its connection with diseases of the Kidneys, Heart, Lungs, and Liver. Third edition, 1858, p. 9. Basham continures, "The ear detects, by the aid of the one, the alterations of the sounds of respiration induced by disease, the eye, assisted by the other, sees in the urine materials and products thrown off from the kidneys, which when carefully studied, become safe and reliable exponents both of the nature of the disease, and of its advance or decline"

an estimate of the progression of the disease process. Basham compares this method of estimating progress of the disease with the then accepted measures, specific gravity or the "weight" of protein or other solids, and finds his use of careful description of the casts under the microscope as equally or perhaps superior to these more established methods.

Continuing along these lines of considering the cell as the basic factor in physiological function as well as pathological changes he states, "It is now universally admitted that the functions of secretion, equally with the process of development and growth, are performed through the agency of the cells... Accordingly we find that in every direction in which microscopic research has been hitherto made, evidence has been obtained of alterations in the character of the cellular elements."[9] He discusses the "healthy" epithelial glands" of the kidney, referring to Mr. Bowman's description of the basement membrane and continues with alterations in "renal disturbance accompanied by albuminous urine and dropsy." He describes and beautifully illustrates changes in epithelial cells in other organs as well. The changes in the composition of the blood, " increase of water and decrease in blood corpuscles" are attributed to these epithelial cell changes. These changes lead to "wide spread decay (in) that the parts and cells which are the seat of it become totally unfit and incapable of ministering to the functions either of nutrition or excretion." He then discussed the

---

[9] Basham, William, Croonian Lectures, 1864, The significance of Dropsy, p.8.

origin of "tube-casts in morbus Brightii" quoting the work of George Johnson.[10]

Basham's enthusiastic acceptance of the cellular basis of function and pathology would seem by current standards overdrawn and stretched beyond the limits of the observations. Basham suggests that the albuminuria of chronic renal disease is a secretion related to the abnormalities of the impaired tubular cells. The concept of glomerulo filtration with protein leakage would need to wait consideration for the future.

How Basham's concepts of importance of nutrition and significance of anemia would modify his suggestions for the treatment of chronic renal disease.

The importance of supporting the epithelial cells of the renal tubules is used in the second Croonian Lecture to alter the current treatment of chronic renal disease. Basham would eschew the treatment of inflammation, the then current standard goal of therapy, at least in the chronic stage of the disease. Rather than bleeding cupping, and purging, etc as his predecessors would advise, Basham suggested that treatment should be directed "mainly to the renovation of the blood and support and maintenance of its cell forming power."[11] This indeed is a welcome relief from the standard of bleeding, use of leeches, cupping, potassium tartrate and depletions therapies of all sort practiced by the predecessors of Basham, Bright, Christian, Osborne, Rayer, etc. (Bright did not

---

[10] Ibid p.33.

[11] Ibid Lecture 11, p. 26.

recommend leeches however.) Consideration of the diet in acute and chronic forms of Bright's disease in this earlier period was hardly recommended and lip service was given to iron therapy or *steel* as it was commonly designated. Diet and iron took on a secondary role to wearing of flannels to avoid chilling, diaphoresis as especially advocated by Osborne, or removal to a warmer or agreeable climate as recommended by Bright, Rayer and even William Osler. Basham substitutes improving the metabolism of cell coupled with correcting the anemia as aims of therapy rather than attack on inflammation. Basham could not free himself however from accepting the then current party line of considering the onset of the disease with its bounding rapid pulse pulse, often fever, and flushed appearance as signs of inflammation, a fire within, needing treatment with depletion therapy, Neither could Basham free himself from the accepted etiology of the condition as related to cold or wet, with alcohol a contributing factor. I t is to be remembered that William Osler accepted these tenants as to etiology and treatment as well.

Basham in reviewing these commonly recommended standards form of treatment rather than dismissing them out of hand, admits they the may be useful in the acute onset of the disease with edema where the features of inflammation may be present. But as the disease progresses attention to the changes in the degenerative changes in the endothelial cells as reflected by examining the urine for casts and the changes in the blood with anemia indicate the need to improved nutrition as well as supplemental iron to correct the anemia and allow the endothelial cells to regenerate. He is firmly against use of bloodletting in this regard.

"Will the abstraction of blood globules from a fluid already exhausted of these, and reduced to a minimum, give aid to renewed cell-growth ? In the acute form of the disease I do not affirm that diaphoretics are not needful. I do not affirm that purgatives are not often most salutary in reducing the amount of fluid accumulated in the tissues. I do not say that digitalis is not a most efficient agent in certain stages of these disorders; but I do say that they are each and all insufficient – positively harmful, if not accompanied or followed, according to their action, by agents and remedies intended to fulfill the fundamental principle of treatment, the restoration of the organism of the power of reproduction of those cells which are rapidly disappearing by processes of solution and decay.

<u>With regard to bloodletting, I unhesitatingly assert that it is injurious: it is manifestly hostile to the fundamental principle on which the treatment of these forms of disease should be based</u>. So long as these disorders were considered as inflammatory, so long as the dropsy was viewed as a product of inflammatory action, such treatment by venesection, or cupping, was only consistent with those doctrines. But here are forms of diseased action in which the blood itself exhibits a deficiency of its most important constituent, in which to take more blood would be but to deteriorate still more the quality of the already impoverished fluid.[12]

Such a strong stand against blood letting at this time was unusual, and seems more emphatic than that of Pierre Louis who in 1825 on statistical basis, *methode numerique*, advocated against bleeding in pneumonia. Even William Osler found bleeding in

---

[12] Ibid, Lecture ll p. 47-48.

acute pneumonia a positive benefit and in renal disease something to consider in his text book in 1892. Basham's acceptance of the microscopic findings of cell change and injury in Bright's disease convinced him that nutritional factors affecting the endothelial cells including improving the anemia were of paramount importance.

Basham continues with a more positive approach to the therapy of dropsy with albuminuria, based on recognition of cellular pathological changes as a clue to need for nutritional and supportive modes of therapy.

Rest, warmth, nutritive stimuli, and blood-forming remedies (haematics) are the agents by which this object may be accomplished.[13]

Here Basham turns the tables on the priority for treatment of dropsy. Considering that inflammation was the root cause of the condition Bright, Christian and Rayer, those who established the clinical entity of Bright's disease, all advocated bleeding and depletion therapies to counter act the signs that were considered to indicated inflammation. Osborne in Ireland advocated initially laxatives then diaphoretic measures such as foot, hip or general baths, followed by Dover pills (Ipecac/Opium) as a diaphoretic agent. Lip service was given to what Basham advocated, rest —no one could argue against bed rest to rest the offending organ, warmth—flannels were advocated by Bright and Christison, primarily to prevent chilling, considered an etiological factor in the condition. Nutritive stimuli – "nutritive food of

---

[13] Ibid, Lecture ll. p. 48.

easy digestion [14]and absence of spirituous liquors" was favored by Christison, but not until after blood letting, leeching, depletion measures, counterirritants, laxatives.

Basham's recommendation for the use of blood-forming remedies (haematics) was either ignored or placed low on list of therapeutic measures by the followers of Bright. While describing pallor, Bright doesn't mention use of iron or other agents[15]. Christison who in a footnote[16] described an elegant but laborious method of estimating *hematosin* and anemia as a factor in chronic renal disease as well as after repeated blood letting, follows Bright in ignoring "blood-forming remedies." He did favor the improving nutrition. Rayer after an array of therapeutic agents, teas, laxatives purgative, Sedlitz or Pullna water, etc, recommends that "when the patients are very weak the harsher purgatives are mixed with ferruginous (iron) agents."[17]   Robert Elliotson's *Principles and Practices of Medicine* a standard textbook of medicine of 1839 in treating the dropsy of renal disease recommends, "here wine and perhaps good nourishment become

---

[14] Elliotson, Robert, Principles and Practice of Medicine, p. 173, 1839.

[15]   Bright, Richard, Cases and Observations, Illustrative of Renal Disease accompanied with the Secretion of Albuminous Urine, Guy's Hospital Repots, vol. 1, 1836. Case 11, "In the month of July 1835, a medical gentleman from the country, aged 33, came to consult me with regard to his general health. His countenance was somewhat pallid; otherwise, his looks did not bespeak material disease."

[16] Christison, Robert, Granular degeneration of the Kidnies and its connection with dropsy, inflammatous and other disease, 1839, p. 32-34.

[17] Rayer, Pierre, Traite des maladies des reins, 1839, p. 150.

necessary, together with steel (iron), sulfate of quinine, and various diuretics."

Basham continues along the same approach he has been advocating. He continues with a list similar to William Osler's conservative approach to management :"**Warmth** is in itself so essential an element of nutrition that it is only necessary for me to observe here, that a careful attention to maintain the surface of the body at an equable state of temperature by means of flannel clothing, and in the winter time by avoiding an exposure to irregularity of cold are advantages which cannot be over estimated in the management of renal dropsy" Here **flannels** and the **avoidance of cold** are justified by their favorable action on nutritive function rather than to prevent relapses of the underlying condition.

Next Basham lists "the influence of **pure air,** the stimulus given to the blood forming power by the agency of pure air, is too well known to require further remark. In the management of cases in a rank of life where **change of residence** can be commanded, the sea-side, or resort to localities elevated in situation and possessing the characters of what is called a bracing quality, should be selected."[18] Basham comments more fully in *On Dropsy,* "The influence of pure air, the stimulus given to the blood forming power by the agency of pure air, is too well known to require further remark. In the management of the cases in a rank of

---

[18] Richard Bright, Pierre Rayer, Willam Osler and others all advocated these general measures, warmth , rest, change of climate, in renal disease but Basham's new twist is the employment of these modalities in the name of improving nutrition or augmenting blood forming.

life where change of residence can be commanded, the seaside, or resort to localities elevated in situation , and possessing the characters of what is called a bracing quality, should be selected. The influence of sea air in the treatment of chronic albuminuria is most potent, and when the means and circumstances o the patient permit, a sea voyage of some duration should be undertaken. A voyage to Australia offers less variability in the extremes of climate than one to India, and is therefore to be preferred."[19] Osler had recommended removal to Southern California for a similar purpose.

Bashan next takes up "nutritive stimulants." He takes up the "controversial" consideration of whether "alcohol is a nutritive element or not." His predecessors especially Richard Bright listed alcohol as a major cause of the disease. Rather he comes down on the side of Rayer who recommended, "daily use of a ferruginous preparation and a small quantity of good white wine."[20]

I will venture to look at it simply from the clinical point of view without committing myself to the declaration, that wine or alcohol is a nutriment. I will venture,

---

[19] Basham, W.R., On Dropsy, and its connection with Diseases of the Kidneys, Heart, Lungs, and Liver, Third edition, 1858. This is to be compared with William Osler in his Principles and Practice of Medicine 1892, p. 709. "A patient in good circumstances may be urged to go away during the winter months or, if necessary , to move altogether to a warm equable climate, lie hate of Southern California.'

[20] Rayer, Pierre, Traite des Maladies des Reins, Tome 2, Nephrite albunineuse p. 156. Translation by Carr, T and Levy, R.I. in progress.

nevertheless, to assert that clinical observation proves it a most efficient (hand-maid) aid to nutritives.---They must be used in moderate quantity, and always in conjunction with food, particularly animal food, either at, or immediately after the meal. They must, on no account, be taken on an empty stomach.--.

It is at this point that Basham begins a discussion of the use of iron and its preparation. "The preparations of iron have long been justly regarded as instrumental in helping to enrich the blood with red corpuscles; and hence appropriately enough called haematemics."

Liquor Ferri et Ammonii Acetatis (Basham's Mixture)

The preparations of iron have long been justly regarded a instrumental in helping to enrich the blood with red corpuscles; and hence appropriately enough called haematics. In all cases where there is evidence of a poor defective blood, called by whatsoever name, anaemia, spanaemia, leukaemia, in the sequel of many acute disease, whether as r\the result of treatment by bleeding, as was formerly the case in acute rheumatic fever, or from the blood-destroying character of the disease itself, as in the convalescing stage of most fevers, whether continued or intermittent, the rapid and beneficial restorative action of chalybeate medicine or steel (chalybeate and steel implies ferrum or iron)[21] *as it is popularly called, particularly in conjunction with animal food and wine, is universally acknowledge and confirmed by daily experience. The preparations of iron in the 'Pharmacopeia' are numerous, but there is one which in these cases of renal dropsy stands pre-eminent*

---

[21] Estes, J. Worth, Dictionary of Protopharmacology 1990, p. 44, 182.

for its efficacy and should be preferred in these cases before all others. It is the tincture of the sesquichloride. (FeCl3)

Thus iron in the form of ferric chloride is the basic ingredient of Basham's mixture. Iron was an ancient history and appears in the Ebers Papyrus from Egypt around 1500 BC[22] as a cure for baldness, invoking the suns ray to charm away alopecia and applying a mixture of iron, red-lead, onions, alabaster and honey. The Bible mentions iron many times but not for medicinal purposes. Pierre Blaud in 1832 demonstrated the use of ferrous sulfate combined with potassium carbonate to improve the low iron content of patients with chlorosis (a form of iron deficient anemia). Blaud treated thirty cases of chlorosis in large doses with improvement. Blaud's pills became a staple of the textbooks.[23] Studies in the early twentieth century have shown that ferrous, the reduced form of iron rather than the ferric form is better absorbed from the duodenum, giving some doubt on the superiority of Basham's mixture. But to continue with Basham, since his mixture contains more that just Ferric chloride.

But it is not as the a sesquichloride that its efficacy is most perceived in these cases. It is as an ammonio-chloride, kept in solution by acetic acid, that its beneficial influence becomes most apparent. It is a very simple preparation, a few drops of the tincture (tincture of the sesquichloride, FeCl3), according to the age of the

---

[22] Bryan, C.P., The Papyrus Ebers 1931. p. 156.

[23] Fairbanks, V.F., Fahey, J.L., Beutler, E., Clinical Disorders of Iron Metabolism,1971, p.15.

patient, are added to a dram of the liquor ammonia acetatis, previously acidulated with acetic acid.

*If this is not done-if the sesquichloride is added to the neutral liquor, an insoluble ammonio-chloride falls, which is with difficulty again taken up; but, if the saline is first acidulated a **beautiful sherry-red fluid** is produced, which is neither unpalatable, nor liable to decomposition and may be kept any time. The tincture of the sesquichloride has long possessed the favorable opinion of physicians in most cases of renal or genito-vesical disorder.*

It is this last paragraph that deserves the most attention. Could it have been that it was that *beautiful sherry-red fluid* that most attracted Basham to his mixture ? The fact that the preparation was soluble and not liable to precipitation, as Blaud's pills were, and that the mixture was *neither unpalatable, nor liable to decomposition and may be kept any time* all add to its advantage. It is to be noted that opinions differ as to its stability and the U.S. Dispensatory 24 edition of 1947 has some reservations in this regard.[24] But it is this last statement of Basham, *The tincture of the sesquichlorid has long possessed the favorable opinion of physicians in most cases of renal or genito-vesical disorder* that is most problematic. No case studies are reported to testify to the effectiveness of this mixture, as was

---

[24] U.S. Dispensatory 24th edition 1947, p. 598. "It should be borne in mind that this was never intended to be a permanent solution, and in time precipitation set in although somewhat retarded by the presence of glycerine. Some pharmacists adopt the plan of keeping all the ingredients, except the ferric chloride tincture and water, mixed together in advance, and when called upon to dispense the solution, to add the proper quantity of tincture and water; this saves time and enables them to dispense a clear solution."

the case with Blaud pills where 30 cases were reported in 1832 on their effectiveness in chlorosis. The U.P.Dispensatory comments on this point as well denying Basham's claim for the mixture, Basham's statement to the contrary.[25] William Olser recommended iron in various preparations in his text book (perchloride, ie: FeCl3 alone, FeI3, Fe(PO4)3 other than as Basham's mixture). I wonder if Osler's recommendation for the use of Basham's mixture which only appears in this chapter on Bright's disease may not have been based on its role as an hematemic, but rather stemming on general principles from the authority of Basham's statement in this Croonian lecture.

Let us again look at Osler's paragraph which mentions Basham's mixture in the very last sentence of the paragraph. Use of iron preparations, without particular choice noted, for anemia is already mentioned several lines above. Basham's mixture is like a parting gesture, a casual throw away thought, a wave to authority. Was Osler equally infatuated with the color, that beautiful sherry red color or was it as noted by Basham that "the tincture of the sesquichloride has long possessed the favorable opinion of physicians ?" Hot baths, acetate of potash, digitalis and a diuretic often a mercurial but with Osler a milder theobromine preparation, were commonly used by Bright and his followers. Osler's recommendation of a low salt diet in contrast was a relatively recent concept in the treatment of

---

[25] Ibid., p. 599." Basham's mixture is used as a hematinic and diuretic and has been popularly employed in chronic Bright's disease. There has arisen a superstition that it exercise a curative effect in nephritis, which its originator, Dr. Basham, never claimed for it."

dropsy, not to be found in the writings of the nascent nephrologists from Bright to Basham earlier in the century.

Indeed the anemia of chronic renal disease is not primarily an iron deficient anemia but it wasn't until 1957 that a hormone produced in the kidney, Erythropoietin, was shown by Jacobson[26] to be the main factor in the anemia of chronic renal disease. (Hemolysis and blood loss are minor factors in the anemia of renal disease. I remember performing chromium tagged red blood cells studies for Dr. C.V.Moore in St. Louis in the early 1950ies demonstrating a mild hemolytic component.) The effectiveness of Erythropoietin has been overwhelmingly demonstrated in the chronic dialysis population, significantly raising the hematocrit. Iron alone is ineffective but in combination with Erythropoietin considerably improves the quality of life of patients with chronic renal failure. Basham as well as William Osler I am sure would have welcomed these results as an improvement on Basham's Mixture.

Summary

Basham acknowledged his indebtedness to Richard Bright for recognizing the relationship between dropsy, coagualable urine and renal disease. He was able to employ the microscope and the concept of cellular pathology to consider more carefully the significance of the tube casts and their possible significance in the understanding of renal disease. Basham, while not able to throw off the concept of

---

[26] Jacobson, L.O., Goldwasser, E. , Fried, W. and Plzak, L., Role of the Kidney in Erythropoiesis, Nature 179, 633, 1957.

inflammation as the initial pathological factor in initiation of renal disease, used his concept of the importance of nutrition and the quality of the blood in the chronic phase to condemn bleeding and other efforts at depletion therapy directed towards inflammation. He recommended an iron preparation, *Liquor Ferri et Ammonii Acetatis* (Basham's Mixture) that remained in the pharmological texts for over one hundred years and made it into William Osler's text as one of the agents in the treatment of renal disease.

Chapter Ten

Nicholas Monardes, Guaiacum—the Holy Wood from the New World, and The French Pox

Dos Libros—Historia Medicinal de las Cosas que se traen de Nuestras Indias Occidentales (1565-1574)

Two Books – Medical History of the Things that are Brought from Our West Indies

Nicholas Monardes

"The New World sent the Old more than gold and ideas. It also confronted Europeans with new animals, from bison to microorganism, and new plants, from tobacco to potatoes."
Anthony Grafton[1]

"The discovery of exotic medicinal plants unknown to European physicians aroused as much excitement then

---

[1] Grafton, Anthony, New Worlds, Ancient Texts, The Power of Tradition and the Shock of Discovery, Belknap Press of Harvard University Press, p.13, 1992.

as the discovery of penicillin did in the 1940s. This is well illustrated by the title given to the English translation (by John Frampton) *of the book in which Nicolas Monardes, a Spanish doctor, first described the most important medicinal plants of America — 'Joyful Newes out of the Newe Found Worlde (1577)'*
F. N.L. Poynter[2]

Following the discovery of the New World by Columbus in 1492, the Spanish followed up their entry on to the American continent with not only a search for gold, silver, and conquering of vast areas of Central and South America but with a keen interest as well in the new animals as well as plants, trees and roots for their use as new foods but also for the potential use of new and unique medicinal products. This paper will review some of these potential medicinal products, emphasizing Guaiacum, as documented by a physician in Seville, Nicholas Monardes, who while never visiting the New World, recorded the vast amount of plants and other items that came through Seville. He recorded his findings in a book entitled, *Dos Libros — Historia Medicinal de las Cosas que se traen de Nuestras Indias Occidentales* (*Two books, Medical History of the Things that are Brought from Our West Indies 1565–1571*).

Nicholas Monardes

---

[2] Two Pioneers of Tropical Medicine: Garcia d'Orta and Nicolas Monardes, introduction by F.N.L.Poynter by C.R. Boxer, Wellcome Historical Medical Library, The Wellcome Building Euston Road, London, M.W. 1 Lecture Series No. 1, 1961.

Who was Nicholas Monardes? He was a physician living in Seville, Spain. Seville was designated as the place where all outgoing ships and incoming material from the New World would be regulated. The House of Trade (Casa de la Contratacion, est. in 1503) supervised these activities under orders of the King, Phillip 11. Monardes would observe the various plants and other materials being brought back form the New World and he interviewed those who had experience with the use of these plants as medications as well as the reports of the native Indian's account of their use of the material. He planted the seeds from many plants in his garden and had an opportunity to observe their effects on his patients. Initially as a young physician he was skeptical of the benefit of certain materials such as *mechoacan*, a root from an area of Mexico, called Michoacan. It was a laxative and alleged to cure a wide variety of conditions. However Monardes was initially cautious in its use since there were no documented reports of its effectiveness or personal experience in its use. However in questioning a variety of people who had testified to its usefulness and gaining experience with the material himself, Monardes eventually devoted a large chapter in this book, *Dos Libros*, to a description of the root, how it was to be prepared and documenting reports of its use and his own experience of its value.[3] According to Antonio Barrera-Osoriom:[4]

---

[3] Knowledge and Empiricism in the Sixteenth-Century Spanish Atlantic World, Antonio Barrera-Osorio, Chapter 11, p. 228 in Science in the Spanish and Portuguese Empires, 1500 -1800, Edited by Daniela Bleichmar, Paula De Vos, Kristin Huffine, and Kevin Scheehan. Stanford University Press, 2009.

[4] Ibid p. 229.

"Monardes continued to write about mechoacan and many other medicinal herbs coming from the New World. He kept asking soldiers, merchants, Franciscans, royal officials and women about new medicines and plants: many brought medicines from New Spain in their luggage, just s modern-day travelers might carry pain-relief and allergy medicines. The doctor asked travelers to provide the names and uses of the substances they brought, and to describe their own experiences using them. Most referred back to Indian uses and Indian names of the various herbs. At some point, he started receiving his own samples of medicines with accompanying reports. Monardes established a botanical garden-and he was not the only one to do so in Seville. He so fully trusted the empirical reports accompanying his samples that he used them without any of the original concerns he had had about mechoacan. On one occasion, he received a medicine said to induce abortions. Knowing only that the Indians used it for that purpose, he tried it in Seville and it worked. Monardes published three reports on these medicines in 1565, 1569 and 1575. The first report ended with these words:

'We are certainly worth a great reprehension for nobody is writing anything about all the herbs and plants from New Spain. Nobody knows anything about their characteristics and shapes to compare them with our own medicines. If someone had the desire to investigate and experiment with so many medicines as the Indians sell in their markets, that would be a thing of great utility and benefit.' "

"Dos Libros"- Two Books and its Translation by John Frampton Entitled, *"Joyfull Newes Out of the Newe Founde Worlde"*

Dos Libros became the most complete and authoritative document of the medical use of plants and other material from the New World in the 16th century translated into Latin, French and English as well as a variety of other languages. The English translation was by John Frampton in 1567 and entitled with the enticing title, *Joyfull Newes Out of the Newe Founde Worlde.* According to C.R. Boxer, John Frampton was " a West Country merchant formerly domiciled in Spain, who had been imprisoned and tortured by the Inquisition before making his escape from Cadiz in 1567 who devoted the rest of his life to translating scientific and travel books from Spanish into English."[5]

Nicholas Monardes and Garcia D'Orta

A contemporary of Mondares, Garcia D'Orta was also a physician but living in Portugal who immigrated to Goa, a Portuguese colony on the west cost of India, and wrote a similar book describing the plants of medical value in the East Indies. His book was entitled, *"Coloquios dos simples e drogas of consas medicinias da India"* (Colloquy of Drugs and Medications of India). d'Orta's book was in the form of a dialogue. C.R. Boxer has compared these two physicians' contributions noting their similarities and differences.[6]

"Monardes described the American species of coca, mechoacan, sarsaparilla and sassafras among others,

---

[5] Two Pioneers of Tropical Medicine: Garcia D'Orta and Nicolas Monardes, C.R. Boxer, F.B.A. , Comoens Professor of Portuguese, Kings College, London, Wellcome Historical Medical Library , 1961, p. 23.

[6] Ibid, p. 23.

while d'Orta described such Asian products as aloes, camphor, candalwood and betel. They both grew up with the concept of humoral pathology as well as unfounded traditions such as the curative properties of the bezoarstone. Both were moderate and sensible in their use of bleeding, purging and dieting. The works of d'Orta and Monardes on exotic material medical complemented and supplemented each other in so many ways, it was fitting that their diffusion throughout the learned world of the sixteenth to seventeenth century Europe was chiefly due to the joint Latin versions of them made by the Flemish physician and botanist, Charles de L'Escluse (1526-1609)"

C.R. Boxer points out however that while d'Orta emigrated to Goa and lived there *his entire life, Monardes never left Spain, gathering reports, interviewing returning* explores about the potential plants that might prove of medical value and gaining experience of there effectiveness in Seville. Dr. Boxer did not feel that either Monardes or d'Orta ever met and that they did there work independently. Also while Mondares was a devout Catholic, d'Orta's parents were Jewish, expelled from Spain in 1492 he was a converso and probably left Portugal for the East Indies for reasons of potential persecution.

Of the Guaiacan, and of the Holie Woodde
Account of Monardes as translated by John
Frampton in *"Joyfull Newes Out of the Newe Founde Worlde"*

Guaiacan was considered the wonder drug of the early sixteenth for the sudden epidemic of what was then called the *French Pox*, later called Syphilus. "Whether the French Pox had existed in

Europe long before, or whether it had recently been imported from America by the crew of Columbus has not yet been decided."[7]   Karl Sudhoff in an essay, *The Origin of Syphilis,* doubted the American origin of Syphilis.[8]

In 1494 Charles the eighth of France leading his forces through Italy toward Naples which fell to the French in February 1495. A devastating epidemic followed which the French called the Neapolitan Disease and the Italians, as might be expected, called the French Disease. It became widely prevalent in Europe, Monardes from this quotation in his chapter *"Of Guaiacum and of the Holie Woodde"*1577 had no question as to the origin of this new disease in Europe, indicating its spread from the New World, its mode of spread or its treatment:

"A Spanyarde that did suffer greate paines of the Poxe, whiche he had by the compaine of an Indian woman, but his servaunte being one of the Phisitions of that countrie, gave unto hym the water of Guaiacan, wherewith many other Spanyardes, that were infected with the same evill were healed verie well of the evill with the whiche many other Spanyardes, that were infected with the same evill were healed, the whiche was thence hether to Sevill, and from thence it was divulged throughout all Spaine, and from thence it was divulged throughout all Spaine, and from thence through all the worlde, for that the infection

---

[7] Tempkin, Owsei, Therapeutic Trends and the Treatment of Syphilis before 1900, Bulletin of the History of Medicine, 29, 1955, p. 309.

[8] Sudhoff, Karl, forward by Fielding H. Garrison, translated by Albert Allemann,   The Origin of Syphilis, in Essays in the History of Medicine, New York Medical Life Press, p.259 – 272, 1926.

wente sowen abroade, throughout all Spaine, and from thence through all the worlde, for that the infection wente sowen abroade through all the worlde, for that the infection wente sowen abroade throughout and surely for this evil it is the beste, and the moste chief remedie of as many as hether unto hath been founde, and with moste assuraunce, and moste certaintie , it healeth this water given as it ought to be, it is certain that it healeth most perfectly, without turnyng to fall againe, except the sicke man doe return to the tumble in the same bosome, where he tooke the firste."[9]

Ulrich von Hutten

While mercury was initially tried in the treatment of the French Pox, the superiority of Guaiacan, a tree from Santa Domingo, an evergreen shade tree with height of 40 – fifty feet, gained favor. It has been called "a gift of the New World to the Old" and a decoction of the wood was popularized by Ulrich von Hutten in 1518 in a very popular widely circulated book, published in Augsburg, *"On the Miraculous Medicine Called Guaiacum Wood, and How to Cure the French Disease" (Die guaiaci medicina et morbo gallico).* Hutten was a German knight, poet, traveler, supporter of the Reformation, who had the disease himself and describes in detail his illness, primarily a skin condition with ulcerations and eventually bony involvement. Hutten in his book states, *"that guaiacum was brought to us from the island Spangnola* (Santa Domingo). *All the inhabitants of the island itself suffer from time to time from the Gallic sickness, as we do from the smallpox. And they use no other treatment against it. A certain Spanish*

---

[9] Monardes, Nicholas, as translated by John Frampton, Joyfull Newes Out of the Newe Founde Worlde, p. 28.

noble when he was governor in the province and was sorely afflicted with the disease itself, shown the treatment by the natives, brought it use to Spain, at first very fearful lest it might not have the same effect across the sea as in the island."[10]

Hutten's Description of His Disease, Preparation of the Wood, and Details of Treatment

Hutten describes in detail the extent and severity of his skin lesions, how the wood is prepared, the rigors of the treatment consisting of not only the drinking of a decoction of the wood, but attempts at humeral treatment consisting of sweating, production of salava, use of laxatives so that "the bowels are made to move by purgative medicine… and being covered up for warmth for a whole hour before he drinks. Food is taken as little as possible…but only to prevent death and sustain life, not to build up strength, and no danger should be feared in this for there is power in guaiacum to build up and strengthen but only in the case of empty stomachs."[11]

Hutten's incisive and dramatic description of his skeletal lesions in chapter 25 of his book on the *Cure of the Gallic Disease* is remarkable as a patient's account of his own condition:

---

[10] Hutten, Ulrich von, The remarkable Medicine Guaiacum and the Cure of the Gallic Disease, translated by Clarence W. Mendell, Archives of Dermatology and Syphilogy, Vol 23, March 1931, number 3, p. 418-19.

[11] Hutten, Ulrich, von, The remarkable Medicine Guaiacum and the cure of the Gallic Disease, published in Mainz 1519, translated by Clarence W. Mendell, Archives of Dermatology and Syphilology Vol 23, March 1931, p. 423.

First my left foot, to which the disease had clung for more than eight years became useless, and in the middle of my tibia, where the least flesh covers the skin, there were inflamed, necrotic ulcers in swollen flesh, causing great pain. When one healed another broke out, for I had many ulcers scattered about, and the skill of no physician could coalesce them into one. Above these there was a swelling as hard as bone and in it immense uninterrupted pain. Just above the right ankle there also was a gathering, also as hard as bone, the oldest remnant of the early stages of the disease. When the physicians tried to remove this with the knife, with fire, and with all sorts of caustics they achieved nothing; but it would now swell violently with the greatest pain and then subside and be more moderate. When I placed my feet near the fire the pain diminished, yet they could not tolerate being covered by many garments. Therefore there was a violent discharge which plainly seemed inexhaustible, and as often as I put weight on my foot it suffered unbearable pain...etc[12].

Hutten had a remarkable initial recovery using guaiacum, following the prescribed regimen and was able to travel extensively thereafter primarily on horseback over large areas of Europe but finally died in a hut on an island in Lake Zurick in 1523 four years after the publication of his book, at the age of 35. The reception of the book gave an overwhelming boost to the use of guaiacum immediately and for the next one hundred years. This in part may have been influenced as well by the Fuggers Company of Augsburg, Germany who were said to have a monopoly on its importation and encouraged its sales and prospered by its use.

---

[12] As translated by Thomas G. Benedek in The Influence of Ulrick Von Hutten's Medical Descriptions and Metaphorical Use of Medicine, Bulletin of the History of Mecicine 66: 3 (1992 Fall) p 362.

Hutton was not the only person to report his experience with "the wood" in the treatment of syphilis. Benevento Cellini the well known Italian goldsmith and sculptor of the 16th century in his autobiography as translated by John Addington Symonds indicates:

Benvento Cellini's Experience with Syphilis

It was true indeed that I had got the sickness; but I believed I caught it from that fine young servant girl whom I was keeping when my house was robbed. The French disease, for it was that, remained in me more than was not like what one commonly observes, but covered my flesh with certain blisters, of the size or sixpences, and rose-colored. The doctors would not call it the French disease, albeit I told them why I thought it was that. I went on treating myself according to their methods, but derived no benefit. ***At last I resolved on taking the wood (this is Guaiacum, called by the Italians Leno santo)*** *against the advice of the first physician in Rome, and I took it with the most scrupulous discipline and rules of abstinence that could be thought of; and after a few days I perceived in me a great amendment.* ***The result was that at the end of fifty days I was cured and as sound as a fish in the*** *water.*[13]   Many authors have tried to explain Cellini's cure of Syphilis, if he indeed had Syphilis, as related to a poisoning with mercury, cure with malaria contracted in the marshlands south of Rome (see footnote 11) and even considering that he had Reiter's syndrome on basis of reports of him having gout.

Other Drugs Used in the Treatment of Syphilis

Compared with the mercury, treatment with guaiacum produced less side effects and the popularity of Hutten's book, with his learning and wit, became the standard of care of the day in the early 16th century. There were some who criticized the treatment with the wood, such as Paracelsus who extolled mercury as the alternative, pointing out measures to avoid the side effects of mercurialism. Paracelsus considered the only miracle of guaiacum was the "growing revenue which it brought to the coffers of the holders of the guaiacum import monopoly, the Fuggers of Augsburg.[14]

---

[13] The Life of Benvenuto Cellini, translated by John Addington Symonds, chapter 59, p. 109, 1951. The next paragraph in Cellini's Autobiography indicates a further use of the wood (Guaiacum). *Exposing myself to wind and water, and to staying out in marshlands I fell a hundred times more ill than I had been before. I put myself once more under doctor's orders and attended to their directions but grew always worse. When the fever fell upon me I resolved on having* **recourse again to the wood (guaiacum); but the doctors forbad it, saying that if I took it with the fever on me, I should not have a week to live.** *However, I made my mind up to disobey their orders observed the same diet as I had formerly adopted and after drinking the decoction for four days, was wholly rid of fever…etc.*

[14] Pagel, Walter, Paracelsus, An Introduction to Philosophical Medicine in the Era of the Renaissance. 1958. p. 24.

Other drugs, soporifics that promoted perspiration, described by Menardes in his book as translated by Frampton renamed, *"Joyfull Newes out of the Newe Founde Worlde"* such as China root, sarsaparilla, and sassafras found temporary favor as supplementary treatment of syphilis as well.

Menardes in his chapter on *"Of the China* indicates that *"it is a root not unlike that described by the Portuguese who brought it to these partes with greate estimation, for to heale all maner of diseases, and especially the disease of the Poxe, in the whiche it hath doen great effects, and the Water is gieven in this forme.The sick person being pourged as is most convenient…etc.*

With regard to the **Sarcaparillia**, Monardes indicates, *"It first came from the new Spaine and the Indians did use it for a great medicine, with the whiche they did heale many and divers disease."* He describes it as a root being a yard long the colour of *"Tawny."* *"I have founde great effects in the infirmities where is suspected the evill of the Poxe, as in large and importunate deseases, the whiche the common remedies of Phisicke hath not profited, although proceaded not of the Frenche Poxe, it dooeth cure and heale theim, as it is seen by the woorke of hym that use it."* Sarcaparilla until recently was a common ingredient in Root Beer.

Sassafras, "Of the Tree that is Brought from the Florida, Whiche is called Sassafras." Menardes indicates that sassafras is a tree found in Florida. *"In the evill of the Poxe, it doeth the same effects that the reste of the water of the holie woodd* (guaiacum), *the China, and the Sarcaparillia dooeth. In the Poxe that bee of a long tyme, it maketh a better and greater woorke, then in them that bee of little tyme.* It was recommended for many other conditions as well.[15]

Naming the Disease: The Poem *"Syphilis Sive Morbus Gallicus" of Girolamo Fracastoro*[16]

Girolamo Fracastoro was a physician, poet with a great knowledge of Latin poetry and Virgil, a philosopher and overall Renaissance Man who became famous for his invention of the name of a disease, *Syphilis,* which until that time had many designations indicating the putative origin or the condition, such as *Morbus Gallicus,* the French Disease. His poem entitled *Syphilis sive Morbus Gallicum,* (Syphilis or the French Disease) was published in 1530. The poem in Latin hexameter, after Virgil's model consists of three books.

The first and second book describes the alleged origin of the disease in America and treatment with mercury. It is in the third book that the poet describes the new remedy, Guaiac or *lignum santi,* beginning with the discovery of the tree in America:

"Sancta arbos, quae sola modum, requiemque dolori,

---

[15] Menardes, Nicholas, Medicinal de las Cosas que se traen de nuestras Indias Cooidentales que siruen en Medicina, 1574, as translated by John Frampton under the title of Joyfull newes out of the newe founde worlde, 1577, Of the China p35 – 37, Sarcaparillia p. 38 -44 (Sarcaparilla was an agent in Root Beer in the past), Sassafras, p. 99 - 120

[16] Much of this portion the paper on Fracastoro's poem on "syphilis" comes from the article by G. L. Hendrickson, Professor of Latin and Greek Literature in Yale University, Bulletin of the Institue of the History of Medicine, vol 2, number 9, November 1934.

Et finem didit aerumnis aerumnis."[17]
(Of the sacred tree which alone has set bounds to
your pain and
Brought our distresses to an end.)

The poet continues with a description of the
preparation and use of the wood, Guiaicum, much
of it taken from von Hutten book, *"The Remarkable
Medicine Guaicum and the Cure of the Gallic Disease"*
The remainder of Book 3 is taken up with the myth
of the discovery of the tree in the New World,
origin of the disease and the remedy of the native
Indians. This is presented in the "atmosphere of
mythical invention against a background of real or
assumed historical fact." [18] A Sheppard, **Syphilus**, is
introduced who is the first to contact the disease,
presenting with hideous sores over the body. A
nymph Ammerice, shows the gathered people how
to cure the condition with gift of the Gods, the tree
Guiaicum sent from heaven. "The original rite of
atonement called for the sacrifice of Syphilus
himself, but Apollo substitutes a bullock as victim
in his stead."[19] (comparison with story of Isaac in
the Hebrew bible is to be noted) "In this story the
ultimate thing which the poet set out to explain
was the origin of the sacred wood guiaicum, but
incidental to that he explains the origin of the
disease and the origin of the name by which it was

---

[17] Syphilis or the French Disease as translated by Heneage
Wynne-Finch, p. 134, line 6and 7.

[18] Hendrickson, G.L., The "Syphilis" of Girolamo Fracastoro,
Bulletin of the Institutue of the History of Medicine, vol 2,
number 9, 1934, p. 526.

[19] Ibid. p. 527.

known. The name syphilis was derived from a postulated imaginary shepherd Syphilus."[20]

It took some time, two hundred years, for the name Syphilis to replace the former names, indicating the putative origin of the disease, such as the French Pox, as can be seen in Shakespeare's *Henry the Fifth of 1600*, Act V,Scene 2, **Pistol:** *News have I that my Neill is dead I'th spital of a* **malady of France**. (spital - hospital)

The Slow Demise of Guaiacum as a Treatment of Syphilis

Unfortunately the dramatic improvement in the condition of Ulrich von Hutten was short lived and he died four years after publication of his book with bone lesions compatible with syphilitic osteomyelitis.

"Physical evidence, in the form of Hutten's skeleton, substantiates his descriptions of his disabilities. Exhumed in 1968, it showed him to have been a small man, about five feet one inch tall. Lesions compatible with syphilitic osteomyelitis were found in the left femur, both tibiae and fibulae, the right ulna, the left humerus.... The deformity of the distal left tibia was consistent with a rigid ankle, his earliest complaint."[21] Studies from the mid twentieth century suggest the rarity of destructive bone lesions in syphilis, only 15

---

[20] Ibid p.528-29.

[21] Benedek, Thomas, G. the Influence of Ulrickvon Hutten's Medical Descriptions, Bulletin of the History of Medicine, 66:3 (1992:Fall) p. 365, quoting Hermann Jung, "Die Lues des Ulrick von Hutten, Hautarzt, 1969, 20: 334-36; idem, Die Lues am Hutten Skelet,

instances of boney involvement from among 10,000 case of early syphilis reported at the Johns Hopkins Hospital in 1942.[22]

Other physicians, Ruiz de Isla, Michael Blondus and Fracastorius in the 16th century all found favor with mercury. Fracastorius whose poem naming the disease as Syphilis initially favored Guiaicum but 16 years later when he wrote *De Contagione* in 1556, hinting at a possible infectious agent describing "seeds of disease and insensible particles", now favored mercury. Jean Fernel the famous French Physician on the other hand advocated guiaicum over mercury "Mercury, Fernel contended, cured the disease in few people, and then only in those who were strong and where the evil was in its very beginning."[23] In 1566 there appeared a summary of published works of over sixty authors, a massive folio in two volumes, by Aloysius Luisinus, *De. Morbo Gallico*, *"serving as a textbook of practical knowledge for the physician of the last half of the sixteenth century."*[24]

The well respected physician, Herman Boerhaave in 1728 reedited Luisinus being very enthusiastic

---

[22] Reynolds, Frank W. and Wasserman, Harry, Destructive Osseous Lesions in Early Syphilis, Arch. Int. Med. 69, 1942, p. 263 – 276.

[23] Temkin, O, The Double Face of Janus, chapter 37 Therapeutic Trends and the Treatment of Syphilis before1900, p.520 quoting Jean Fernel, *Le meilleur traitement du mal venerien,* transl.l L. Le Pileur, Paris, 1879, p.88.

[24] Zimmermann, E.L., Texts and Documents, Early collections of Syphilologic Works, Aloysiou Luisinus and His Influence on Syphilogy, Institute of the History of Medicine, Bulletin 4, p598, 1936.

on the use of Guiaicum. He recommended its use in the preface to *"Aphrodisiacus sive de lue venereal"*: *"Must, then the venereal patient, who by nature of his illness, cannot be helped with quicksilver, be given up as hopeless? By no means ! What, therefore, can be done to help when mercury is ineffectual? I will tell. Read Hutten's tract inserted here, but reread it with care; you will see that the most intricate contagion can be washed away by the sharp elixir of guaiacum."*[25]

The Frenchman, Jean Astruc published a weighty compendium and review *"Treatise on the Venereal Disease"* in Latin consisting of six books in 1737, translated by William Barrow into English. He championed the American etiology of Syphilis but recommended mercurial unction as safer and more effective than Guaiacum but the latter still had its place is some cases. He questioned "Might not Guaiacum when freshly cut down and full of Sap, be possessed of the Virtue in Hispaniola, which it wants in Europe, where it is administered dry and withered."[26] Thomas Sydenham even earlier in 1717 in his chapter on *Treatise on the French Pox*, again preferring the older designation to Fracastoro's *Syphilis*, expressed similar reservations, "not withstanding what we say of the great Virtue of Guaiacum and Sarsaparilla in the places where they grow which are thought in a manner to lose their virtue in the long passage to us."[27]

---

[25] Munger, Robert S. Guaiacum, the Holy Wood from the New World, Journal of the History of Medicine 4 (1949) p. 219.

[26] Ibid, p. 220

[27] Sydenham, Thomas, The whole works of that excellent practical physician, 1717, Treatise on the French Pox, p 246-265.

With the development of the printing press in the mid fifteenth century, medical reports and printed manuscripts in the 16th through the 18th centuries on this newly recognized disease popularized *morbus gallicus* making information and treatment more available than in the past. Gradually the original name of the disease, French Pox, lost favor to Fracastoro's Syphilis and Guiaicum as well lost favor in its treatment, although was still mentioned as an alternative treatment in some Pharmacopeias of the nineteenth century.

The use of Guiaicum as adjunctive therapy was reported by Jonathan Pereira as late as 1846 in his massive compendium, *The Elements of Materia Medica and Therapeutics*. Pereira, from the Royal College of Physicians in London gives some history of the drug's introduction into Europe in the early 16th century, 1508, from the natives of Santo Domingo. He describes in detail the parts of the tree for medicinal use, the bark, resin or gum, and the wood itself. The uses of Guaiacum are listed: chronic rheumatism, gout, chronic skin conditions, as well as a remedy for venereal disease which he indicates *"was at one time in great repute."* Quoting Nicholas Poll he indicates that, *"within 9 years from the time of its introduction into Europe more than 3000 persons had derived permanent benefit from its use."* Regarding its current use he indicates, **"Experience, however, has taught us the true value of the remedy and we now know that Guaiac has no specific powers in curing or alleviating syphilis. It is applicable, as an alternative and sudorific for the** *relief of secondary symptoms, especially venereal rheumatism and cutaneous eruptions..*[28]

Guaiacum did make a recovery in the twentieth with a phenolic compound derived from the resin of the Guaiacum tree which was used universally to detect blood in the stool when a blue color was produced by the addition of hydrogen peroxide.

Conclusion

While the American origin of Syphilis has always remained a controversy, the enthusiastic recommendation of Hutten and the popularity of Mondares book describing the vast number of plant products of medicinal value that he cataloged from his base in Seville, including the chapter *"On Guaiacum and the Holie Woodde"* paved the way for *Guaiacum* to be the agent of choice in the treatment of the great epidemic of the French Pox that ravaged Europe at the end of the 15th and early 16th centuries. *"As Guaiacum was considered a specific antidote for syphilis and as it came from America, it followed that the disease came from America also. Certainly of all the exotic remedies used through the centuries in the treatment of the greatest of all social diseases, none was more lauded, and at the same time less efficacious that the holy Wood from the New World."*[29] Arsenicals and eventually Penicillin, not until the 20th century, were found to be more effective treatment when the causative agent,

---

[28] Pereira, Jonathan, The elements of Materia Medica and Therapeutics, 2nf American Edition , 2 volumes (Philadelphia, Lea and Blanchard, 1846, 2 p. 638-640.

[29] Munger, Robert S. Guaiacum, the Holy Wood from the New World, Journal of the History of Medicine 4 (1949, , p 229,.

Treponema palllidum and more specific diagnostic tests became available.

Summary

Nicholas Monardes a physician who never left Spain used his home city of Seville which was the port of entry of large quantities of plants and other products to record and evaluate potential agents of medicinal value.

In his book, *"Dos Libros, Medical History of Things that are Brought from Our West Indies"* 1565-1571, he described among many items, including Guaiacum, a tree the wood of which was said to be effective in the treatment of the French Pox that ravaged Europe in the late 15th and 16th centuries.

Ulrich von Hutten's book, *"The Remarkable Medicine Guiacum and the Cure of the Gallic Disease"* was universally initially accepted and touted as a cure for this epidemic.

While the American origin of the of Syphilis has remained a controversy, its treatment with Guaiacum had a brief dramatic acceptance in the 16th century as an agent in its cure with its use lingering over the next several centuries.

Guaiacum became an agent that was abundantly accepted and praised but ultimately proved to be a worthless, in the Epidemic of the French Pox that sweep Europe in the late 15th and 16th centuries.

Afterword[1]

The Imperative of Physicians to life save and heal

David B. Levy, PhD, MLS

The question regarding the relationship of G-d as Healer[2] versus the physician's prerogative to

---

1 The afterword is greatly indebted and cites widely from the article, "The Obligation to Heal: The Right and the Obligation of the Physician to Heal" compiled by Rabbi Zvi Ilani & Rabbi Yaakov Weinberger, translated from the Hebrew by Uriah F. Cheskin & Yitchak Pechenick; appears in Jewish Medical Ethics, vol 2 by the Dr. Falk Schlesinger Institute for Medical-Halachic Research, Jerusalem: 2006.

2 Sources that imply that Healing is Only the divine prerogative include: (1) God healed Avimelech (Gen 20:17); For I am G-d your Healer (Ex 15:26); I will remove illness from your midst (Ex 23:25); Please God please heal her (Numb 12:13); I have smitten and I will heal (Deut 32:39); Cure me God and I will be healed (Jer. 17:14); I will restore health to you and I will heal you of your wounds (Jer 30:17); For he makes sore and binds up (Job 5:18); Heal me G-d for my bones shudder (Ps. 6:3); O Lord my God I cried to you and you have healed me (Ps. 30:3); The healer of all your diseases (Ps. 103:3); He sends His word and HE heals them (Ps. 107:20); He heals the broken hearted (Ps. 147:3).

heal[3] give rise to many grey areas in Jewish law but derives *deoreita* from Biblical sources (*and*

---

[3] Sources which indicate that Healing is the Physicians prerogative are: (1) And man became a living soul (Gen 2:8); Rabbi Yossi explains: Sustain the soul which I gave you (Taanit 22b); (2) He shall pay for his victims period of incapacitation and he shall cause him to be thoroughly healed (Ex 21:19). Rabbi Ishmael said: this verse contains the authorization for physicians to heal (Berachot 60a; Bava Kama 85a); (3) "observe my laws and my judgements which if a person does he shall live through them (Lev 18:5); (4) A physician who heals and sustains a patient is fulfilling the mitzvah of maintaining bodily health contained in this verse (Rabbi Solmon ben Aderet Sefer Isssur V'hetter, ch. 60, sect 8-9); (5) Do not stand idly by the blood of your brother... and you shall love your neighbor as yourself (Lev 19:16,18)... this verse requires a physician to provide medical assistance to save and ease the pains of a sick person who is suffering or in danger (Responsa Tzitz Eliezer pt. 15, sec 38); (6) And your brother shall live with you (Lev 25:36) The physician who heals the body of a sick person or relieves his body of suffering, fulfills the mitzvah (Sefer Issur v'hetter loc cit); (7) Take great head for yourselves (Deut 4:13) The physician who heals a sick person fulfills the mitzvah contained in this verse (Sefer issur v'hetter loc cit); (8) If you see your neighbor's ox or his sheep straying do not close your eyes to them. You shall surely return them to your borther... and return it to him... and so shall you do for every lost item belonging to your brother which he loses and you find (Deut 22:1-3). The Plain meaning of the verse refers to returning a lost item. But from the repetition of the words "Return them" and "return it to him" Hazal interpret the verse is referring also to a return of his body to health (Sanh 73a); (9) You may not hide yourself (Deut 22:3). Just as the finder of a lost object is not permitted to ignore it, but must take the trouble to return the object to its owner(s) so must a physician return lost bodily capacity to the patient by curing his malady. He must not try to evade his responsibility and hid from the sick person (Responsa Tzitz Eliezer loc cit).

thou shalt love your neighbor[4] and *not stand idly by their blood (al takmod dam reakhah)* and *DeRabanna* from Rabbinic texts.

A question is asked what is the source, and from where does *the permission to heal* and *the imperative* to assist in healing derive in the Bible and Rabbinic texts? The two conditions permission, and imperative are not the same terms in meaning. Permission assumes that G-d is the real Healer, and the physician merely a conduit to enabling G-d's healing via knowledge of the laws of nature to be manifest. Some Rabbis like The Chida and Ramban note that one should not totally rely on the healing methods of a physician because only G-d is the true Healer.

---

[4] See H. Cohen, *Der Religion der Vernunft: Aus den Quellen des Judentums*, "The Discovery of Man as Fellowman (mitmensch), and "The Problem of Religious Love", Leipzig, 1918.; Rosenzweig's discussions of love of God and love of enemies in notes on poems of Yehudah Halevi, love letters to his wife Edith Hahn, the role love plays with regards to Revelation (*Offenbarung*) in *Die Stern der Erloesung*; Hannah Arendt's dissertation on *Liebesbegrieff bei Augustin* (Love and Saint Augustine, Chicago: University of Chicago Press, 1996), Scholem's *Mysticism*, 233-5; Buber's *Ich und Du* and *Between Man and Man* 28-30, 51-58; Leo Baeck's *Das Wesen des Judentum*, Berlin, 1936, p. 193; For example Cohen writes, "Und der Mensch liebt Gott. Aber dass der Mensch Gott liebt, is praktisch und psychologisch nicht schlechtin die Umkehrung von der Liebe Gottes zum Menschen. Es muss noch eine doppelte Vermittlung hinzukommen, um die Liebe des Menschen zu Gott vermitteln. Der Mensch muss erstlich den Mitmenschen lieben. In dieser Liebe, welche die Sozialpolitik erzeugt, liegt der wahre Grund der Menschenliebe, Und nur von diesem Grunde aus kann der Gedanke enstehen, dass auch der Mensch zur Liebe Gottes sich erheben könne. Er kann ja den Mitmenschen lieben. Und wie konnte er dies, wenn ihm Gott nicht in dem heiligen Geiste in dem Geiste der Heilikeit den Geist der Liebe in Herz gelegt hatte (*Der Religion der Vernunft*, Leipzig, 1918, p.478)

The sources for permission and the imperative to heal are multiple but one that attributes the "cause" of injury to human action is in Exodus 21:18-19

וְכִי-יְרִיבֻן אֲנָשִׁים--וְהִכָּה-אִישׁ אֶת-רֵעֵהוּ, בְּאֶבֶן אוֹ בְאֶגְרֹף; וְלֹא יָמוּת, וְנָפַל לְמִשְׁכָּב.

18 And if men contend, and one smite the other with a stone, or with his fist, and he die not, but keep his bed;

יט אִם-יָקוּם וְהִתְהַלֵּךְ בַּחוּץ, עַל-מִשְׁעַנְתּוֹ--וְנִקָּה הַמַּכֶּה: רַק שִׁבְתּוֹ יִתֵּן, וְרַפֹּא יְרַפֵּא. {ס}

19 if he rise again, and walk abroad upon his staff, then shall he that smote him be quit; only he shall pay for the loss of his time, and shall cause him to be thoroughly healed.

The text requires that anyone who strikes another person, in this case a pregnant women, to cause the victim to be healed, and if the child in the womb is miscarried the perpetrator of the miscarriage is liable not only for the potential loss of life to the women but also to her potential offspring.

RAMBAM (1135-1204)

There are many sources for the imperative to heal and one is the commandment not to stand idly by the blood of one's neighbor.[5] The obligation to heal according to Rambam is found in multiple places.

לֹא תַעֲמֹד עַל דַּם רֵעֲךָ 5

In the *Pirush al ha-mishnah on Nedarim* 4:4[6] the Rambam holds healing is obligatory:

The Law requires the physician to heal Jews. This is part of what they said in the Talmud when they explained that the verse "you shall surely restore it to him[7]" includes the obligation to heal the sick. For if you see someone being harmed and you can save him, you are to save him with your body, with your property, or with your knowledge.

For the Rambam physicians must or are obligated to use their know-how, their skill, and experience to provide medical care for just as the verse "*you shall surely restore it (health) to him*" obligates the returning of lost objects, so too the physician is obligated to return to patients lost health by restoring it. The Rambam references Deut 22:

לֹא-תִרְאֶה אֶת-שׁוֹר אָחִיךָ אוֹ אֶת-שֵׂיוֹ, נִדָּחִים, וְהִתְעַלַּמְתָּ, מֵהֶם: הָשֵׁב תְּשִׁיבֵם, לְאָחִיךָ.

1 Thou shalt not see thy brother's ox or his sheep driven away, and hide thyself from them; thou shalt surely bring them back unto thy brother.

---

6 המודר הנאה מחבירו ונכנס לבקרו עומד אבל לא יושב ומרפאהו רפואת נפש אבל לא רפואת ממון ורוחץ עמו באמבטיא גדולה אבל לא בקטנה ויישן עמו במטה רבי יהודה אומר בימות החמה אבל לא בימות הגשמים מפני שהוא מהנהו ומיסב עמו על המטה ואוכל עמו על השלחן אבל לא מן התמחוי אבל אוכל הוא עמו מן התמחוי החוזר לא יאכל עמו מן האבוס שלפני הפועלים ולא יעשה עמו באומן דברי רבי מאיר וחכמים אומרים עושה הוא ברחוק ממנו:

7 Deut 22:1-2

ב וְאִם-לֹא קָרוֹב אָחִיךָ אֵלֶיךָ,
וְלֹא יְדַעְתּוֹ--וַאֲסַפְתּוֹ, אֶל-תּוֹךְ
בֵּיתֶךָ, וְהָיָה עִמְּךָ עַד דְּרֹשׁ אָחִיךָ
אֹתוֹ, וַהֲשֵׁבֹתוֹ לוֹ.

2 And if thy brother be not nigh unto thee, and thou know him not, then thou shalt bring it home to thy house, and it shall be with thee until thy brother require it, and thou shalt restore it to him.

The concept of property is transformed to health in general in Maimonides formulation reasoning *"if we must save or restore lost property kal ve-homer, minor ad majoris, we must also restore or save life."* In the above verses from Deuteronomy the Talmud says that this means the obligation of the physician who must save an endangered life.[8] Rambam also codified the law of lifesaving elsewhere in *Hilchot Rotseach* 1:14.[9] For Rambam the physician's obligation to heal is part and parcel of the commandment of lifesaving in general which in turn derives from the obligation to return lost property. If for instance someone is drowning on Shabbat, the laws of Shabbat are suspended due to *pekuah nefesh* to save the person in the water. Likewise a *gemara in Yoma 85a* legislates that if a building has fallen on someone on Shabbat subsequent debate arises to how much one may remove the rubble (a forbidden work on Shabbos) either to the nose (Gen 7:22) (respiration), the mouth (respiration), or the heart (cardiac function) which plays a central seminal textual role in the

---

[8] Sanhedrin 73a

[9] כל היכול להציל ולא הציל עובר על לא תעמוד על דם רעך. וכן הרואה את חבירו טובע בים. או ליסטים באים עליו. או חיה רעה באה עליו. ויכול להצילו הוא בעצמו. או ששכר אחרים להצילו ולא הציל. או ששמע עובדי כוכבים או מוסרים מחשבים עליו רעה או טומנין לו פח ולא גלה אוזן חבירו והודיעו. או שידע בעובד כוכבים או באונס שהוא בא על חבירו ויכול לפייסו בגלל חבירו להסיר מה שבלבו ולא פייסו וכל כיוצא בדברים אלו. העושה אותם עובר על לא תעמוד על דם רעך

criteria for determining brain death in rabbinic law. The principle affirmed is that life is sacred and the imperative of life saving, even on Shabbos.

RASHBA, (Spain 1235-1310)

The Rashba also held that medical practice is obligatory but for different reasons. In a Responsa[10] the Rashba evokes that a patient is prohibited from endangering themselves by "relying on a miracle." He evokes the Talmudic case of a leaning wall which is said to remind one of their sins.[11] Further the Rashba marshals *Taanit* which asserts, "Anyone who relies on a miracle will not be granted a miracle.[12] Only extremely righteous and saintly persons can be saved by a miracle.[13] Even the most pious may not rely on G-d in the course of their endeavors unless they act in accord with the laws of nature. They may not say, "I shall fill my candle with water or wine" and rely on a miracle to ignite it. Of course someone like Eliyahua ha-Navi did exactly that. Eliyahu directed cisterns of water to be filled on Har Carmel and a fire from heaven came down and ignited them still in the face of the Baal prophets that Eliyahu put to death. The Rashba is therefore saying that after the era of prophecy the sick, even the most righteous, must apply the rules of nature which the physician knows, to try to be

---

10 Responsa, 1:413

11 Berachot 55a

12 Taanit 20b

13 For example, with regard to Rabbi Chanina ben Dosa and wild animals, Hazal state, "Woe to the man who encounters a wild animal, as they said, woe to the wild animal which encounters Rabbi Chanina ben Dosa" (Berachot 37a. If a venomous snake bit Rabbi Chanina the snake would die.

cured and not rely on the miraculous change of nature. The sick must not refrain therefore from therapy. Even if the person suffers because of *yisurin shel ahava* (sufferings brought on to cause them to repent out of love) they should keep in mind "if your walls are dangerously leaning, remember your sins!." Although some sin more than others, no one except a newborn is free from sin. Thus according to the Rashba the patient is obligated to accept treatment.

CHIDA (Rabbi Chayim Yosef David Azulai)
(1724-1806)

The Chida followed the Rashba but added a formulation to support the patients obligation to accept medical treatment.[14] The Chida notes that "nowadays" one should not rely on miracles. This is because of the *yoredet* in history that each subsequent generation is less meritorious or farther from Sinaitic revelation. The Chida evokes the idea of "common practice." The Chida argues that the pious of old who did not need physicians are on a *medrega* that is not that of today of even the most righteous. He notes that it would be prideful to equate one with those previous *tzadikim*. He remarks that it is common practice to accept healing by physicians. However he urges the sick to cling to the Creator to strengthen His mercy with all their heart as trusting only in Him. As the dollar states, "in God we trust"! The Chida is skeptical and identifies as prideful those who refuse treatment in the belief that G-d will miraculously heal them as they place themselves in the exalted company of the most pious of old who were

---

14 Birchei Yosef, Yoreh Deah 336:2

worthy of miracles. It is more realistic to have a more modest view of oneself. While all *poskim* hold that ultimately the source of healing is G-d, they recognize that the physician can be an emissary or vehicle through whom G-d's healing can transpire in part. The pusek "have him thoroughly healed[15]" implies that the Torah permits the physician to heal. The Chida underscores that reliance soley on miracles is "almost prohibited" but he acknowledged that in part such reliance is a good impulse and not prohibited in essence because it accepts G-d's omnipotence. The Chida reasons that 'nowadays" when such miracles are rare, it would be chutzpah for any individual to consider themselves worthy of an open miracle that changes laws of nature.

RAMBAN (Spain, 1194-1270)

The Chida rejects the more radical opinion of the Ramban. While like Rambam, Ramban was a physician, they differed with regard to the healing power of the medical art. In the Ramban's commentary on the Torah on Leviticus 26:11 which states:

וּפָנִיתִי אֲלֵיכֶם--וְהִפְרֵיתִי אֶתְכֶם, וְהִרְבֵּיתִי אֶתְכֶם; וַהֲקִימֹתִי אֶת-בְּרִיתִי, אִתְּכֶם.	**9** And I will have respect unto you, and make you fruitful, and multiply you; and will establish My covenant with you.
י וַאֲכַלְתֶּם יָשָׁן, נוֹשָׁן; וְיָשָׁן, מִפְּנֵי חָדָשׁ תּוֹצִיאוּ.	**10** And ye shall eat old store long kept, and ye shall bring forth the old from before the new.

וְנָתַתִּי מִשְׁכָּנִי,	**יא**	**11** And I will set My tabernacle
בְּתוֹכְכֶם; וְלֹא-תִגְעַל		among you, and My soul shall
נַפְשִׁי, אֶתְכֶם.		not abhor you.

וְהִתְהַלַּכְתִּי, בְּתוֹכְכֶם,	**יב**	**12** And I will walk among you,
וְהָיִיתִי לָכֶם, לֵאלֹהִים;		and will be your God, and ye
וְאַתֶּם, תִּהְיוּ-לִי לְעָם		shall be My people.

When the children of Israel do the will of G-d then the L-rd blesses their bread and their water and removes all illness from their midst[16] so they have no need of physicians and no need to protect themselves by any medical strategies as it is written in Exodus 5:26:

וַיֹּאמֶר אִם-שָׁמוֹעַ	**26** and He said: 'If thou wilt
תִּשְׁמַע לְקוֹל ד'	diligently hearken to the voice of the
אֱלֹהֶיךָ, וְהַיָּשָׁר	LORD thy God, and wilt do that
בְּעֵינָיו תַּעֲשֶׂה,	which is right in His eyes, and wilt
וְהַאֲזַנְתָּ לְמִצְוֹתָיו,	give ear to His commandments, and
וְשָׁמַרְתָּ כָּל-חֻקָּיו--	keep all His statutes, I will put none
כָּ ל - הַ מַּ חֲ לָ ה	of the diseases upon thee, which I
אֲ שֶׁ ר - שַׂ מְ תִּ י	have put upon the Egyptians; for I
בְמִצְרַיִם, לֹא-אָשִׂים	am the LORD that healeth thee.'
עָלֶיךָ, כִּי אֲנִי ד',	
רֹפְאֶךָ. {ס}	

Thus the text states "I am the L-rd that healeth thee." Which implies that when the righteous in the times of prophecy fell sick they did not seek physicians but sought out prophets. This is the case with Hezekiah who when he fell sick he was advised by the prophets to pray, and indeed due to his supplication he lived another seven years. It is attested in the medical literature that praying lowers the blood pressure and people who pray, meditate, or play music often live longer. The Ramban holds that the L-rd watches over *Klal*

---

[16] וַעֲבַדְתֶּם, אֵת ד' אֱלֹהֵיכֶם, וּבֵרַךְ אֶת-לַחְמְךָ, וְאֶת-מֵימֶיךָ; וַהֲסִרֹתִי מַחֲלָה, מִקִּרְבֶּךָ
(Shemot 23:25)

Yisrael and heals their ills as long as they obey His mitzvoth. In the days of prophecy to be healed one sought out prophets rather than physicians to be healed for prophets offered religious instruction to bring one closer to G-d who is the ultimate source of healing. In the times just after the Hurban Rabbi Yochanan ben Zakai in asking three things of the emperor Vespacian when Rabbi Yochanan was clandestinely carried out alive in a coffin (*Gitin* 56a-b and *Avot de Rabbi Natan*) to meet the Roman sieger of Jerusalem, requested a physician to cure Rabbi Tzadok. Rabbi Tzadok was starving himself in mourning for the Beit HaMikdash only permitting himself to eat fruit juices. Apparently the close of prophecy and sealing of the Hurban, left a state where even rabbi Yochanan appealed to a physician to cure the righteous Rabbi Zadok. So too all the more for those living later, we should not relie on the miracle caused by a prophet to heal us. While the patient must trust in Hashem always at this time in history one must consult physicians instead of prophets, for the physicians knowledge and skills, at a time where the vast majority are not meritorious to benefit from open miracles changing the laws of nature. After the Hurban and end of prophecy it is common practice to draw on the knowledge of physicians for healing. In Torat ha-Adam the Ramban prohibited practitioners from healing however unless they were qualified and there was no one greater to defer.[17] In Torah ha-Adam the Ramban a second time discusses the ethical status of medical treatment.[18] The Ramban bases himself on Yoma 82a that lifesaving is taught

---

[17] HD Chevel Ramban, p.43-44; Also see D Margalit, Chachmei Yisrael ke-Rofeim.

[18] HD Chevel, Ramban, p.42

at all costs and thus physicians have permission to heal. He thus gives the example of physicians who are experts that a patient should eat on Yom Kippur if in serious danger. Thus he who suffers faintness from fasting is fed honey or sweets until his eyes become clear. These patients are fed on the advice of experts. Ramban notes "he who is quick to provide medical treatment is praise worthy." If a physician refuses to order a patient in danger to eat on Yom Kippur it is as if "he is a spiller of blood" and renouncing of the obligation of lifesaving. Thus when medical practice is permissible it is part of the imperative of lifesaving. Since very few individuals are worthy of miraculous changes in laws of nature and the Torah does not depend on miracles, it is advisable to accept medical treatment from experts. Rav Ovadia, former chief sefardic rabbi of Israel, agrees with the Ramban that "nowadays" in the post-prophetic era medical treatment and therapy is obligatory.[19]

Rabbi Avraham ibn Ezra (1089-1164)

Ibn Ezra Appears to be more strict than others with regards to physicians and life saving. In his commentary on Exodus 21:19 which states:

אִם-יָקוּם וְהִתְהַלֵּךְ	**19** if he rise again, and walk abroad
בַּ ח ו ץ ,	upon his staff, then shall he that
עַל-מִשְׁעַנְתּוֹ--וְנִקָּה	smote him be quit; only he shall pay
הַמַּכֶּה: רַק שִׁבְתּוֹ	for the loss of his time, and shall
יִתֵּן, וְרַפֹּא יְרַפֵּא.	cause him to be thoroughly healed.

Ibn Ezra comments:
כי האמת להשען ישר דרך על בוראו ולא על בינתו, כן
בדרך המזלות ובדרך הרפואות, כי הכתוב אמר: אני ד'

---

[19] Responsa Yehavve Daat 1:61

רופאך (שמות טו, כו), **ואין צורך לעשות רופא אחר שותף עמו**. וכן אמר: והסירותי מחלה מקרבך (שמות כג, כה). וברך את לחמך ואת מימיך (שמות כג, כה). והפך זה: אשר לא תוכל להרפא (דברים כח, כז), גם בחליו לא דרש את ה' כי אם ברופאים (דהי"ב טז, יב), וכן כתוב: מחצתי ואני ארפא (דברים לב, לט), כי הוא יכאיב ויחבש (איוב ה, יח). וטעם ורפא ירפא - מבנין הכבד הדגוש. ואיננו כמו הקל. והמכה היא מיד האדם, ויוכל האדם לרפאותה, ומי ירפא שיכה השם? רק הכתוב אמר: יך ויחבשנו (הושע ו, א). וטעם אשר לא תוכל להרפא (דברים כח, כז) - כאשר תרפא ממכת בן אדם:

Ibn Ezra cites the pusek "I am the L-rd who heals you[20]" and comments And there is not need to do healing other than this by a partner such as a physician. Ibn Ezra notes that it was only Rabbi Ishmael or one Talmudic sage who permitted medical care carte blanche.[21] Ibn Ezra implies there is no need for G-d who is self sufficient and is the Healer of all to make a physician His partner.
Exodus 15:26 reads:

כו וַיֹּאמֶר אִם-שָׁמוֹעַ תִּשְׁמַע לְקוֹל ד' אֱלֹהֶיךָ, וְהַיָּשָׁר בְּעֵינָיו תַּעֲשֶׂה, וְהַאֲזַנְתָּ לְמִצְוֹתָיו, וְשָׁמַרְתָּ כָּל-חֻקָּיו--כָּל-הַמַּחֲלָה אֲשֶׁר-שַׂמְתִּי בְמִצְרַיִם, לֹא-אָשִׂים עָלֶיךָ, כִּי אֲנִי ד', רֹפְאֶךָ. {ס}

26 and He said: 'If thou wilt diligently hearken to the voice of the LORD thy God, and wilt do that which is right in His eyes, and wilt give ear to His commandments, and keep all His statutes, I will put none of the diseases upon thee, which I have put upon the Egyptians; for I am the LORD that healeth thee

Ibn Ezra comments:

---

[20] Ex 15:26   וַיֹּאמֶר אִם-שָׁמוֹעַ תִּשְׁמַע לְקוֹל יְהוָה אֱלֹהֶיךָ, וְהַיָּשָׁר בְּעֵינָיו תַּעֲשֶׂה, וְהַאֲזַנְתָּ לְמִצְוֹתָיו, וְשָׁמַרְתָּ כָּל-חֻקָּיו--כָּל-הַמַּחֲלָה אֲשֶׁר-שַׂמְתִּי בְמִצְרַיִם, לֹא-אָשִׂים עָלֶיךָ, כִּי אֲנִי יְהוָה, רֹפְאֶךָ

[21] Bava Kama 85a

יש לך לזכור, כי בעיניך ראית המחלה והנגעים והמכות
אשר שמתי במצרים בעבור שמרדו בי ואם תשמע חקי
תמלט מהם, שלא אעשה לך כאשר עשיתי להם. ועוד,
כי אני ה' אהיה רופאיך מכל מחלה שגזרתי להיותם על
הארץ[22], אין לך צורך לרופא, כאשר רפאתי המים
המרים, שאין יכולת ברופאים לרפאם.

Ibn Ezra unlike Rambam and Ramban, distinguishes between diseases caused by man, and those caused by G-d. The Torah according to Ibn Ezra permits only physicians to heal with regards to man-made problems. However illness caused by G-d are to be healed only by God.

The Tashbets (Rabbi Simon ben Zemach Duran (1361-1444) rejects ibn Ezra's *makmir* position.[23] For the Tashbets not only is rejecting medical treatment (like the Jehovah's witnesses) folly but it contradicts Jewish law. Other more recent Poskim reject ibn Ezra's strict position in the name of the Ramban, that permission to heal is in fact permission and imperative to fulfill the commandment to heal[24] as long as there is trust in G-d and one believes that everything is from His

---

[22] ... You must remember that you have seen with your own eyes the illness and the blows and the plagues which I have placed upon Egypt due to their rebellion against Me. But if you obey My laws, you will escape them and I shall not do to you as I did to them.... Further "I am the L-rd your Healer."- you will need no physician for any disease which I have decreed to be upon the earth as I curred the bitter waters which no physician could cure.

[23] Responsa Tashbets 1:51

[24] Ramban in Torat ha-Adam

will and a physician his shaliach.[25] Rabbi Yoel Sirkes (the Bach, 1561-1640) expresses a view similar to Rabbi Moss, that if the patient with a divinely inflicted wound turns solely to physicians rather than to G-d...medical treatment is prophibited... but if the patient trusts in God He will send him a remedy... and it is permissible to seek medical treatment even from a divinely inflicted illness.[26] The Bach adds this is the practice of all Jewish communitites. Thus ibn Ezra's view is a minority position. Most poskim with varying spectrums of differentiation hold that lifesaving supersedes all prohibitions of healing. Questions may arise however what about a patient who is not righteous (does not qualify for a miracle to save herself) but they want to reject medical advice to eat prohibited foods? Another classic question regards a sick person or pregnant women to eat on a fast days such as Yom Kippur, ie. How does one ascertain if they are really at major risk?[27] The classic case is referenced in Yoma where the sages say one may not be too strict. The sages said even in a patient says, "I do not need to eat" and the physician says, "He needs to eat", we follow the

---

[25] Rabbi Moshe Mat Moss, Mateh Moshe, Bikkur Cholim 4:3 (= p.221b n Warsaw edition 1876).

[26] Bayit Chadash, Yoreh De'ah 336:1

[27] The case arises of Rabbi Shmuel Bornstein's son-in-law who was very sick. He probably had influenza in the fall of 1916. Although his physician thought it important for him to eat and drink he did not want to comply. Rabbi Bornstein wanted to follow the position of Ramban or Rabbi ibn Ezra to fast on YK against medical advice, thereby being conformity with his father-in-laws father (rabbi A Bornstein of Sochaczew) and his father in laws grandfather(Rabbi Zev N Bornstein of Biale).

physicians advice.[28] One is commanded to open their ears to the words of the Sages even if it appears to be against your particular individual view of Biblical law.[29] Some poskim[30] marshal on the docket the pusek from Koheleth in regards to eating on YK: "Go eat your bread with enjoyment, and drink your wine with a merry heart, for God has already approved what you do."[31] According to Midrash Bamidbar this verse was spoken by a divine voice in the days Shlomo HaMelekh when they ate on Yom Kippur during the construction of the Beit HaMikdash Rishon.[32]

From the above desiderata it is clear that serving as a physician in Judaism fulfills the mitzvah of preserving and restoring life as a shaliach of G-d to benefit mankind and it is for this reason that physicians like Maimonides preferred to earn his *parnasa* via serving as a doctor rather than taking a salary for teaching torah. Rambam cites Pirke

---

28 Yoma 83a. Dr. Kadish via Dr. Fishbane once asked me to find mikorot on the topic: "is a patient allowed to demand that her pacemaker be taken out, even if the doctors know that the prognosis is that she will not live long with it out under her directives. In this sheilah not only is Yoma 83a relevant but the whole topic of the prohibition of euthanasia in Jewish law, for according to Rabbi David Bleich such an order by a patient is like choosing euthanasia for themselves.

29 Zevachim 29a

30 See Shem mi-Shemuel Mo'adim; Rabbi Shmuel wrote against being overly righteous on fasting on YK if one's life is at risk and insisted that his son-in-law follow the physicians instructions.

31 Koheleth 9:7; לֵךְ אֱכֹל בְּשִׂמְחָה לַחְמֶךָ, וּשֲׁתֵה בְלֶב-טוֹב יֵינֶךָ: כִּי כְבָר, רָצָה הָאֱלֹהִים אֶת-מַעֲשֶׂיךָ.

32 Midrash Bamidbar 17:2

Avot[33] that anyone who uses the torah to dig, will be buried by the torah, and it is the Rashba who encouraged Jewish men to go into medicine as an honorable profession for doing good, lifting essentially the bans by certain rabbis from studying the sciences that resulted in the wake of the Maimonidean controversy.[34] Overall serving as a physician who can save lives in partnership (shituff) with G-d is as if the physican helped establish the world for the Mishnah in Sanh states:

**וכל המקיים נפש אחת מישראל מעלה עליו הכתוב
כאילו קיים עולם מלא ומפני שלום הבריות**

Indeed this sentence adorns Sinai Hospital's lobby in Baltimore, and many hospitals throughout the Jewish world, because whoever saves one life is as if they had saved the entire world(s). Such a principle speaks to the power of the physician to do good on behalf of humanity,

---

[33] Pirke avot 4:5

בי צדוק אומר: אל תפרוש מן הצבור, ואל תעש עצמך כעורכי הדינין, ואל תעשה עטרה להתגדל בה, ולא קרדום לחתוך בה; וכך היה הלל אומר: ודאשתמש בתגא, חלף. הא למדת, כל הנהנה מדברי תורה, נוטל חייו מן העולם.

[34] Levy, David B., **Censorship** of Rambam's "Sefer Madda" and "Moreh ha-Nevukhim," Association of Jewish Libraries: Annual Convention 35 (2000) 172-17.

fulfilling Jewish law[35] of which kidney organ donation[36] is just one such modern miracle we are witnessing today,[37] but raising many ethical words of caution as we move into a new world of transhumanism.[38]

For topical bibliographies and mikorot packates prepared by DBL in Medical Halakhah such as: *organ transplants, stem cell research, genetics, taking medicine on the Sabbath and Pesah, brain death controversy, euthanasia prohibition,* on the library

---

[35] See Halperin, Mordechai, Halperin, Mordechai, Medicine, Ethics & Jewish Law 2 (1996) 15-24 ; Siev, Michael, Saving lives : are there limits?, Journal of Halacha and Contemporary Society 62 (2011) 100-119

[36] Boas, Hagai, Organ donation, brain death, and the limits of liberal bioethics., Bioethics and Biopolitics in Israel (2018) 258-275; Prager, Kenneth, Non-heart-beating organ donation : the ethical challenges involved., Halakhic Realities (2015) 107-113; Shabtai, David, Donation after cardiac death : halakhic perspectives., 289-263 (2012) 4 ורפא ירפא; Hashiloni-Dolev, Yael, The regulation of preimplantation genetic diagnosis for sibling donors in Israel, Germany, and England : a comparative look at balancing risks and benefits., Kin, Gene, Community (2010) 61-83; Eisenberg, Daniel,1946-, Organ and tissue donation., Assia - Jewish Medical Ethics 6,2 (2008) 4-12; Scott, Ori, Implementing presumed consent for organ donation in Israel : public, religious and ethical issues, IMAJ 9,11 (2007) 777-781; Finci, Shachar, The potential for organ donation in a university hospital in Israel, IMAJ 5,9 (2003) 615-617;

[37] Mackler, Aaron L., Respecting bodies and saving lives : Jewish perspectives on organ donation and transplantation, Cambridge Quarterly of Healthcare Ethics 10,4 (2001) 420-429.

[38] Schweid, Eliezer, Humanism, globalization, postmodernism, and the Jewish people., The Responsibility of Jewish Philosophy (2013) 97-157; Tirosch-Samuelson, Hava, In defense of Jewish humanism, Jewish History 3,2 (1988) 31-57

guides for- (a) Jews in Medicine, (b) Science and Torah, (c) Jewish Ethics, etc.[39]

---

[39] See (1) http://libguides.tourolib.org/ld.php? content_id=17201576 (2) http://libguides.tourolib.org/c.php? g=114144&p=743034 (3) http://libguides.tourolib.org/c.php? g=114144&p=743100 (4) http://libguides.tourolib.org/c.php? g=114183&p=742870 (5) http://libguides.tourolib.org/ld.php? content_id=17196419 (brain death)

Bibliography

Robert I. Levy, M.D.

Papers Written While in Medical School
(1949-1953)

1. Dissimilation of glucose-1 phosphate and of fructose 1-6 phosphate by isolate rat diaphragm and by cell free effluent from rat diaphragm: K.L. Zierler, R.I. Levy, and R. Andres. *Bulletin of the Johns Hopkins Hospital*, 82:7, 1953.

2. On the mechanism of action of alpha-tocopheryl phosphate with special reference to carbohydrate metabolism of striated muscle.

    a. Effect on the capacity of rat diaphragm to dissimilate hexose phosphate: K.L. Zierler, R.I. Levy, H.M. Anderson and J. L. Lillenthal. *Bulletin of the Johns Hopkins Hospital*, 92:32, 1953.

b. Inhibition of insulin induced glycogenesis on isolated rat diaphragm. K. L, Zierler, R.I. Levy, J.L. Lillenthal. *Bulletin of the Johns Hopkins Hospital,* 92, 41, 1953.

Papers Written during Nephrology Fellowship with Dr. Gilbert H. Mudge (1955-1957)

3. The effect of acid base balance on the diuresis produced by organic and inorganic mercurials : R.I. Levy, I. M. Weiner, and G. H. Mudge. *Journal of Clinical Investigation,* 37: 1016, 1958.

4. Studies on mercurial diuresis: renal excretion, acid stability and structure activity relationships of organic mercurials: I. M. Weiner, R.I. Levy, and G. H. Mudge. *Journal of Pharmacology and Experimental Therapeutics,* 138: 96, 1962

Papers Written During House Staff Training or Medical Practice (1959–2002)

5. Renal failure secondary to ethylene glycol poisoning: R.I. Levy. *Journal of the American Medical Association,* 173, 1210, 1960.

6. Steroid blocking agents as diuretic agents: R.I. Levy. *Sinai Hospital Journal,* 10:110, 1961.

7. Serum sodium concentration: Facts of Fancy: R.I. Levy. *Indian Medical Journal,* 1962, (October).

8. Lipids of the kidney, Blood and Urine in the Nephrotic Syndrome: R.I. Levy, *Fifteenth Annual Conference on the Kidney* 1964.

9. Antibiotics and Digitalis Administration in Uremia : R.I. Levy. Editorial – *Maryland Medical Journal*, 13, 1964.

10. Ethacrynic Acid in Pulmonary Edema: R.I. Levy, A.I. Mendeloff, D. Turner. *American Journal of Clinical Nutrition*, 18: 20, 1966.

11. Studies in a Patient with Chyluria: R. I. Levy, A.I. Mendeloff, D. Turner. *American Journal of Clinical Nutrition*. 18:20, 1966.

12. Overwhelming Salicylate Intoxication in an Adult: R. I. Levy. *Archives of Internal Medicine*, 119, 1967.

13. Treatment of Hypercalcemia with Forced Saline Diuresis and Ethacrynic Acid. R.I. Levy, *Proceeding of the American Society of Nephrology*, 3rd Annual Meeting Washington, D. C. (Abstract) 0.40, 1969.

14. Clinical Spectrum of Lactic Acidosis. R.I. Levy, K. Dharmasena (Paper presented at Regional Meeting, American College of Physicians in Baltimore, MD, October, 1975.

15. Serum Chloride Analysis, Bromide Detection and the Diagnosis of Bromism: *American Journal of Clinical Pathology*, R.I. Levy, R.E. Wenk, Lustgarton, Pappas and Jackson. Vol. 65: 49, 1976

16. Ectopic ACTH, Prostatic Oat Cell Carcinoma and Marked Hypernatremia, R.E. Wenk, B.S. Bahagavan, R.I. Levy, D. Miller and W. Weisburger. *Cancer*, Vol. No 2, August , 1977.

17. Chyloperitoneum in a Peritoneal Dialysis Patient. American *Journal of Kidney Diseases*. Vol 38. No. 3 (Sept) 2001; pE 12.

Articles in Retirement

Mozart and Medicine at the End of the Eighteenth Century   R.I. Levy   1990 Presented at Sinai Hospital Lectureship, Baltimore, MD

Papers Written Following Retirement from Medical Practice, 2002

18. History of Sinai Hospital of Baltimore Maryland 1863 - 2009, Its Place in the History of Jewish Hospitals in America

19. William Osler's Mention of Basham's Mixture in the Treatment of Bright's Disease

20 The Animal Chemists in the Circle of Richard Bright

21. Therapeutic Spectrum Available to Defining the Newly Recognized Clinical Entity: Bright's Disease

22. The Reception in Britain and on the Continent of Richard Bright's – Report of Medical Cases on Linking Dropsy, Coagulable Urine and Small Granular Kidneys as a Clinical Entity

23. A Garland of Ibids: the Use of Footnotes in the Medical Writings of Early Nineteenth Century Authors Who Established Bright's Disease a Clinical Entity

Operate on both Bach and Handel for Cataracts with Disastrous Results ?

32. William A. Marburg's Contribution to Sir William's Osler's Love for books and Libraries

33. Brahms and Billroth: The Musical Composer and Physician- A Musical Friendship

34. Diagnosis of Handel's Ophthalmological Complications: The state of Ophthalmology at the time of Musician Fredrick Handel in the area of cataract surgery

35. William Harvey's *De Motu Cordis*

36. Homer Smith's Philosophy of Evolution and the Evolution of the Kidney

37. Verdi's Opera Falstaff and Otello: Adaptation from Shakespeare's plays, Beyond Similarities and Difference between the Shakespeare plays and Verdi Opera Towards a Vision of the Interplay between Literature and Music

38. Sources of Mozart's *Le nozze di Figaro*

39. Marshmallow Extract as Therapeutic Pharmakon Salve in Homer's Epic the Iliad

40. Medical Remedies Discovered in the New World During Age of Exploration: More than Tomatoes, Corn, and Tobacco

41. A meditation on the portrait of Thomas Kennedy of Hagerston Maryland at Sinai Hospital

who played an important role in the Jewish right to vote

42. The source of an opera by Claude Debussy (L. 88, Paris), Pelleas *et Melisand based on the literary work of Maurice Maeterlinck*

43. *Olivier Messiaen's   Quatuor pour la fin du temps, a musical offering to a Jewish friend in the concentration Camps during the Shoah*

44. *Tribute to David Macht author of* Bones and Verdure. An Appreciation of Science in Biblical Expressions *and* The Heart and Blood in the Bible

45. Kierkegaurd's Fear and Trembling and the Akedat Yitchak

46. Miscellany on Medicine, Science, Music, and the Medical Humanities

Book Reviews

Journal of the History of Medicine and Allied Sciences, Review of: *History of Nephrology 4: Reports from the Third Congress of The International Association for the History of Nephrology.* Basel Switzerland, S. Karger AG, 2002 vi. 218 pp. illus.